The Complete Book of
Home Remedies
for Your Dog

The Complete Book of Home Remedies for Your Dog

Deborah Mitchell

A Lynn Sonberg Book

St. Martin's Paperbacks

The information in this book is not intended to replace the advice of a veterinarian, who should be consulted in matters relating to your pet's health, especially if your pet has existing medical conditions. Individual readers are solely responsible for their own decisions related to their pet's health. The author and the publisher do not accept responsibility for any adverse effects individuals may claim that their pet experiences, whether directly or indirectly, from the information contained in this book.

The fact that an organization or web site is mentioned in the book as a potential source of information does not mean that the author or publisher endorse any of the information they may provide or recommendations they may make.

THE COMPLETE BOOK OF HOME REMEDIES FOR YOUR DOG

Copyright © 2013 by Lynn Sonberg Book Associates.

All rights reserved.

For information address St. Martin's Press, 175 Fifth Avenue, New York, NY 10010.

EAN: 978-1-250-02627-9

Printed in the United States of America

St. Martin's Paperbacks edition / May 2013

St. Martin's Paperbacks are published by St. Martin's Press, 175 Fifth Avenue, New York, NY 10010.

10   9   8   7   6   5   4   3   2   1

Table of Contents

Introduction

For many people, accepting a dog into their household is like welcoming a new member to the family—and, like all family members, they need love, attention, and nurturing. A dog is also a responsibility. Dogs get sick, just as people do . . . and they often require assistance from their human family to help them get better and stay healthy.

WHY HOME REMEDIES FOR DOGS?

As more and more people take charge of their own health by using nutrition, herbal remedies, supplements, and other natural approaches, it makes sense to do the same thing for the four-legged members of the family.

As with your own health, there are some very compelling reasons to turn to home remedies for your dog. For example, Michael knew that cleaning his dog's teeth regularly was important for Reggie's oral health and overall health as well, but he wanted to take control of Reggie's dental care at home. So Michael learned how to clean Reggie's teeth using safe, natural ingredients and using a breath freshener that he makes using parsley. Michael not only keeps Reggie's teeth and gums in good shape but also avoids costly veterinary bills.

When Audrey's cocker spaniel mix, Crackers, developed atopic dermatitis (an itchy skin condition) for the third summer in a row, she decided not to go the usual conventional medicine route and opted to try home remedies. Using a combination of omega-3 fatty acid supplements and switching to a homemade diet, Crackers got through the summer and beyond with minimal scratching, and she didn't need medications and so avoided their side effects. Audrey was happy because Crackers felt better, and she didn't have high vet bills.

Here are a few of the benefits of having home remedies at your fingertips:

- **They provide peace of mind.** When you know which home remedies can provide relief when certain symptoms or health situations arise, you will feel more confident that you'll be able to care for your dog quickly and easily using ingredients or items that are either already in your home or readily available at a neighborhood store.
- **They are cost-effective.** Home remedies can save you money because they are typically more inexpensive than prescriptions or vet visits. In fact, some home remedies—such as apple cider vinegar for ear infections, baking soda for kidney problems, and parsley for the gums—cost only pennies per dose.
- **They minimize or eliminate side effects.** Natural home remedies can reduce or eliminate your dog's exposure to drugs or other treatments that can cause side effects or negative reactions.

The home remedies offered in this book—from the dietary suggestions to the nutritional supplements, herbal remedies, and more—help promote and support the body's ability to heal itself. In some cases the remedies may be used along with conventional treatments offered by your veterinarian. This integrative approach is a more balanced way to support the body's healing process.

Quite honestly, there are very few double-blind, placebo-controlled studies that support the use of natural supplements and remedies to treat canine ailments to back up their use. What we do have, however, are many years of clinical experience from veterinary professionals from around the world, combined with anecdotal reports from happy pet parents, and evidence extrapolated from studies of supplements and natural remedies taken by humans. Fortunately, dogs and humans share many of the same health challenges, and what researchers have learned about treating people sometimes can be extrapolated to apply to dogs. And so man can also be a dog's best friend when it comes to findings ways to improve their health and quality of life.

YOU ARE YOUR DOG'S HEALTH ADVOCATE

Your dog can't buy her own food, get rid of intestinal parasites, cure her own ear infection, or drive herself to the vet. You are your dog's health advocate, which means you are responsible for taking care of your canine companion using conscientious nutrition along with tried-and-true home remedies when she is not feeling well.

A growing number of veterinarians, like many people doctors, have adopted a holistic approach to caring for their patients, and that approach includes techniques beyond traditional vaccinations and medications, such as herbal remedies, special diets people can prepare at home, acupuncture, and nutritional supplements. Similarly, an increasing number of pet parents (I will use this phrase throughout the book rather than "pet owner") are receptive to and want to learn more about home remedies for their dogs.

The immune systems in dogs and in people have amazing powers to promote self-healing. However, those powers can fade rapidly if nutrition is poor and/or if situations arise that compromise the immune system, such as an injury, infection, or disease. That's where you, as your dog's health advocate, come in: by providing him or her with the nutrition necessary to support and maintain health, home remedies to take care of situations that can be handled with love and care at home, and the wisdom to know when to seek help from a professional.

HOW TO USE THIS BOOK

This book is divided into two main sections. Part I is "Canine Cuisine and Nutrition," and it's first because it's the most important. Dogs are like people: Good nutrition is the foundation of sound health, and poor food choices can both cause and exacerbate symptoms, illness, disease, and poor quality of life.

Chances are, you know which foods you should be eating (even if you choose not to eat them), and you have access to a myriad of sources and professionals who can provide sound nutritional advice. But your dog depends on you. She cannot drive to the pet store or prepare her own food. She cannot do the research to make sure they are getting food that meets her nutritional needs. That's part of your responsibility as your dog's health advocate.

How much do you know about dog food? You may be aware of the old expression "I wouldn't feed that to my dog." Well, a variation of that sentiment—"I *shouldn't* feed that to my dog"—applies to much of the commercial dog food on the market. Therefore, the chapters in the "Canine Cuisine and Nutrition" section tackle the issue of how to feed your dog in the most healthful, convenient, and cost-effective manner, addressing questions such as what is in commercial dog foods, how to choose healthful commercial dog foods, and how to prepare economical homemade food for your dog (including recipes). We also provide an appendix listing foods and beverages you should *not* give your dog.

Part II, "Canine Conditions and Home Remedies," will

tell you where you can find detailed information about the most common ailments and diseases that affect dogs, including symptoms, which breeds are more susceptible to the complaint, and how it is typically treated. Each entry also explains which home remedies may help and how you can work with your veterinarian or on your own to apply them.

Veterinarians generally agree that to be a good dog health advocate, you should provide your dog with a nutritious diet and regular exercise, take your dog for a checkup at least once a year, have her teeth cleaned at least once a year (while also brushing her teeth regularly at home in between), and use preventive tick and flea methods.

If you are among the many pet parents who don't meet all of these recommended goals, you are not alone. However, that does not mean you don't want to provide the best you can for your dog. This book can serve as a tool to help you be a better health advocate for your dog when it comes to nutrition and managing common health challenges when they arise and providing home remedies that meet those needs.

PART I

Canine Cuisine and Nutrition

You may wonder why, in a book about home remedies, we are starting out with three chapters on nutrition and diet. After all, isn't that what commercial dog foods are for: so you don't have to worry about what to feed your dog? Can't your dog get all the nutrients he or she needs from any of the dozens—no, scores—of different types and brands of dry, moist, and canned dog foods on the market?

Well, not really. Feeding your dog the types of food that will support, promote, and maintain his health is not as simple as tearing open a big bag and filling his bowl twice a day, although the pet food makers would like you to believe it can be that easy. Actually, it *can* be that easy, but easy isn't necessarily the best for your dog's health. If you are willing to expend just a little bit more effort, your dog will be repaid every day with better health, more energy, and better quality of life, while you can enjoy a happier dog and lower vet bills.

Your dog's diet is a critical part of her overall health and well-being, which is why we have dedicated three chapters to cover what you should know as your dog's health advocate. These chapters include nutritional information, tips, and recipes that are a critical part of the foundation of your dog's health. This information works in tandem with the home remedies that will help promote, support, and maintain your dog's health and assist in preventing or minimizing health challenges that may come her way.

Let us warn you that there are many points of view among veterinarians, pet nutrition experts, and enthusiasts when it comes to what they consider to be the best way to feed your dog. Makers of low-grade dry dog foods will defend their products, but so do the owners of fast-food restaurants and makers of the high-fat, high-sugar, preservative-laden foods on the shelves of supermarkets everywhere. Just because a company makes a product, slaps a label on it, hires marketing agencies to say the ingredients are safe, and puts it on the market doesn't mean it's good for the consumer, whoever he or she is. And that includes your dog.

So the information we offer in these chapters—and throughout this book—is for you to contemplate, digest, research further as you desire, and then act on as you see fit as your dog's health advocate.

Chapter 1

Basic Nutrition: What Your Dog Needs

Providing a safe, nutritionally complete diet is the most important thing you can do for your dog's health. Sound nutrition is the foundation of your dog's well-being. Before you fill up her bowl, whether it's with kibble, canned food, or homemade dog food, it's your responsibility to know which nutrients she needs for optimal health and how much protein, fat, carbohydrates, and different vitamins and minerals are necessary to safeguard her from illness and disease and keep her happy and functioning at the top of her game.

That's the goal of this chapter: helping you learn what your dog needs in her bowl.

YOU, YOUR DOG, AND DINNER

Dogs have lived alongside humans for at least fifteen thousand years (and some experts say twice as long), and over those millennia, the more domesticated dogs became, the more the food they ate resembled that of their two-legged companions. Although our early ancestors ate meat, at least half of their diet was grains, fruits, vegetables, and seeds. The same is generally true today.

Like humans, dogs need a variety of macronutrients (carbohydrates, fats, proteins), vitamins, minerals, and other nutrients, and they can come from a wide assortment of foods—not just from a bag of kibble, from which there's a good chance your dog is not getting the nutrients she needs.

Before I talk about the foods your dog can enjoy in her diet for optimal health, energy, and quality of life, let's look at the specific nutrients that are important for your dog's health.

NUTRIENTS EVERY DOG NEEDS

When you want to know how much vitamin C you should get each day or what the recommended amount of protein is for you or your child, you can turn to the guidelines established by the U.S. Department of Health and Human Services and the U.S. Department of Agriculture. You can also look at the nutritional information available on every package of food you buy. But where do you turn when you want to know about your dog's nutritional requirements? Who is the authority?

The National Academy of Sciences has set standards for specific nutritional requirements for dogs. In addition, the Food and Drug Administration (FDA) regulates pet food, requiring that it be "safe to eat, produced under sanitary conditions, contain no harmful substances, and be truthfully labeled." Standards for dog food manufacturers have been established by the Association of American Feed Control Officials (AAFCO) and its Canine Nutrition Expert Subcommittee. Because the area of commercial dog food is a large and complex one, a fuller discussion of this topic is found in chapter 2.

As you may already know from your knowledge of human nutrition, experts have identified the recommended daily allowances for different nutrients based on the minimum amounts necessary to maintain good health, and this same concept applies to dogs as well. However, each dog is unique, and so your dog's nutritional requirements will depend on his age, size, breed, presence of any health problems, amount of exercise he gets, whether he is taking medications, and other factors.

That said, you need a nutritional foundation to help you identify which nutrients your dog needs. That's what is discussed below, along with explanations of what how each of the nutrients can help support and maintain your dog's health.

Protein

Dogs need protein, whether that protein is in the form of animal-based foods, plant-based foods, or both. (Yes, dogs can thrive on a well-planned vegetarian diet. More on that later.) Protein is critical for your dog's growth and development, as well as to make sure the immune system functions optimally. Your dog's body burns protein as calories and also converts it to and stores it as fat.

Of the twenty-two amino acids that make up protein and that dogs need, your four-legged companion can make twelve of them. The remaining ten are called essential proteins because it is essential to get them from the diet. They include arginine, histidine, isoleucine, leucine, lysine, methionine, phenylalanine, threonine, tryptophan, and valine. If your dog does not get enough of any of these essential amino acids, he can become ill. High-quality proteins contain a healthy balance of all ten of the essential amino acids dogs need.

Some sources of protein are better than others, and that's because each one contains different amounts and different kinds of amino acids, plus each protein source differs in how well the body can break it down into amino acids. The ability of the body to use protein and its amino acids is the biological value. At the top of the list of biological value is the egg, with a value of 100. Milk and fish have a value of 92, while beef is around 78 and soybean meal is 67, meat and bone meal and wheat are about 50, and corn is 45. (Note: Corn and corn products are common ingredients in commercial dog food.) Animal parts such as feathers and hair are also used as protein sources, but they are even lower on the biological value scale.

How much protein does your dog need? Although every dog is different, the general consensus is that puppies need more protein (28 percent of calorie intake) than do adult dogs (18 percent), while nursing dogs need the same as puppies. Experts note that dogs are well equipped to digest and utilize diets that contain higher amounts of protein, although there's no agreement on exactly how much protein is considered to be "too much." If you feed your dog a balanced diet (as discussed in chapter 3, "What's for Dinner: Good Food for Your Dog"), then giving him too much protein should not be a concern.

If you were to give Sparky excessive amounts of protein, his body would use some as calories, convert some into fat, and eliminate some in his urine. If Sparky has any kidney problems, a high-protein diet would not be recommended because it would place too much stress on the kidneys. It is a myth that a high-protein diet will cause kidney disease in dogs. However, your veterinarian may recommend you limit Sparky's protein intake if he had a severe kidney problem (see chapter 12, "Kidney Problems").

Carbohydrates

Carbohydrates are an important energy source for your dog, and they come in the form of starches, cellulose (fiber, which is discussed below), and sugars, and the food sources are primarily vegetables and grains. In commercial dog foods, starchy carbohydrates add form and texture to dry foods, which could not exist without carbohydrates. Canned dog foods can be made without the addition of carbohydrates.

Carbohydrates consist of absorbable carbs, which include glucose and fructose. They are absorbed directly by your dog and don't need to be broken down (metabolized) by enzymes. Digestible carbohydrates are easily metabolized by enzymes, and these carbs include starches and dietary fibers that pass through the small intestine into the colon, where they are fermented by organisms into short-chain fatty acids and gases.

Fiber

Fiber is found in carbohydrates and is available in two forms, although all sources of fiber contain some of each form in varying percentages:

- **Insoluble, which means it does not dissolve in water.** Insoluble fiber gives plants their structure, and it is especially helpful in helping move food through the intestinal tract. Foods that contain a high percentage of insoluble fiber include wheat bran, root vegetable skins, whole grains, brown rice, and carrots.
- **Soluble, which means it does dissolve in water.** Good sources of soluble fiber include barley, beans, fruits, oats, peas, and vegetables.

Experts have not determined exactly how much fiber dogs need, but a reasonable range for adult dogs appears to be 2.5 to 4.5 percent of their daily dietary intake. Scientists do know, however, that a dog's digestive tract is short, which means it is designed more for a carnivorous diet, which typically does not contain lots of fiber/carbohydrates. That said, there are some situations in which feeding your dog some additional fiber is beneficial. For example, dogs who have diabetes (see chapter 8, "Diabetes") can benefit from extra fiber in their diet to help manage blood sugar levels. If your dog is overweight, some additional healthy fiber in her diet can help her feel full without adding pounds (see chapter 13, "Obesity").

Fats

Your dog needs fats in her diet because they provide the most concentrated source of energy from her food. Dogs are able to process and utilize many common fats and oils, including those found naturally in meat, poultry, fish, vegetables, and grains, as well as those added to commercial dog foods, such as poultry fat, cottonseed oil, and tallow. However, not all of these fats are considered to be healthy.

How much fat does your dog need? That depends on factors such as her size, age, level of activity, and breed, but generally puppies need a minimum of 8 percent and a maximum of 17 percent of their total daily calories as fat. Adult dogs who are not doing vigorous exercise (for example, as a sled dog would) need 5 to 15 percent of their daily calories as fat in their diet.

In addition to acting as a fuel source, fats perform other important roles for your dog. For example, they carry fat-soluble vitamins A, D, E, and K throughout the body, make your dog's food taste good and have a desirable texture, and help keep her coat shiny and healthy. The essential fatty acids (such as omega-3 and omega-6) are called essential because they must come from the diet, as your dog cannot make them herself. The essential fatty acids are important for cell structure and function, boosting the immune system, clotting blood after an injury, and keeping your dog's skin and fur healthy.

Among the essential fatty acids, your dog needs omega-3 and omega-6 in his diet. The omega-3s include alpha-linolenic acid (ALA), eicosapentaeonic acid (EPA), and docosahexaenoic acid (DHA). The omega-6 fatty acids include linoleic acid (LA), gamma-linolenic acid (GLA), dihomo-gamma-linolenic acid (DGLA), and arachidonic acid (AA).

The recommended ratio of omega-6 to omega-3 fatty acids your dog needs is between 10:1 and 5:1. Essential fatty acids can be found primarily in cold-water fish, fish oils, vegetables oils (e.g., sunflower and safflower), and some plants. Commercial dog foods typically contain much more omega-6 than omega-3. If you make your own dog food, you may need to add omega-3s as a supplement, depending on the recipes you use.

Too much fat in the diet, however, can result in an overweight dog. Many commercial dog foods contain more fat than recommended and are of poor quality. When dog foods are stored in high heat and humidity, as they often are when being transported or warehoused, the fats in the food can become rancid and the fatty acids can break down. Rancid fats can destroy vitamins A and E and linoleic acid, which can cause a deficiency in these important nutrients.

Vitamins

Dogs need many of the same vitamins you do. Here's what you need to know about vitamins for your dog:

- **Vitamin A.** This vitamin is found in the yellow pigment of plants. Unlike cats, dogs have the ability to make their own vitamin A from carotene, which is found in vegetables, so veggies high in carotene (e.g., carrots, sweet potatoes, and squash) should be a part of your dog's diet.

  Vitamin A is a critical nutrient for the proper growth and development of puppies, but the need for vitamin A doesn't stop there, as it is also essential throughout a dog's life for healthy skin and fur, night vision, and strong muscles. As an antioxidant, vitamin A may help protect against cancer in dogs.

  Vitamin A is a fat-soluble nutrient, which means the fat cells hold on to it and stores it so your dog doesn't need to get the vitamin in every meal. The recommended minimum dose of vitamin A for dogs is about 2,225 IU per pound of food eaten daily or 50 IU/lb of body weight. Although excessive amounts of vitamin A can cause abnormal bones and muscle weakness, you would have to give your dog extremely high doses of vitamin A for a long time before these complications occurred.

- **Vitamin B complex.** The B family of vitamins is found in meat and vegetables and is important for growth and for nerve support, function, and regeneration. Dogs who are deficient in B vitamins can experience reflex problems, diarrhea, hair loss, eye problems, heart failure, and loss of appetite.

  Because the B vitamins work synergistically, they should be taken as a complex if you use a supplement, unless your veterinarian instructs you otherwise. Typically, a multivitamin/mineral supplement for dogs contains the B vitamins. (See "Supplements for Dogs" on page 21.) The B vitamins are water soluble, so your dog will eliminate any excess B vitamins in her urine.

  The minimum requirement for each of the B vitamins is as follows:

  ✓ Thiamin (B_1): 0.01 mg/lb
  ✓ Riboflavin (B_2): 0.05 mg/lb
  ✓ Niacin (B_3): 0.12 mg/lb
  ✓ Pantothenic acid (B_5): 0.1 mg/lb
  ✓ B_6: 0.01 mg/lb
  ✓ Folic acid: 0.002 mg/lb
  ✓ Biotin: 0.001 mg/lb
  ✓ B_{12}: 0.00025 mg/lb

- **Vitamin C.** Under normal conditions, dogs can produce their own vitamin C, so there is no recommended daily dose. However, dogs who are under stress (e.g., as a result of pregnancy, being in a kennel, illness, or emotional trauma such as separation anxiety) may need additional vitamin C to make up for what their body cannot produce. Since vitamin C is water soluble, your dog will eliminate any excess vitamin C in her pee if you give her too much, so don't worry about a vitamin C overdose (although diarrhea may occur).

- **Vitamin D.** Like humans, dogs produce their own vitamin D from the sun, but they also get it from their diet in foods such as liver and fish oils. Vitamin D is essential for dogs to help the body retain calcium for strong bones and teeth, and it also plays a critical role in muscle and nerve control. Veterinarians often recommend puppies be given a vitamin D supplement to support their growth and development. If your dog is on a vegetarian diet, you should give him a vitamin D supplement. The minimum recommended amount of vitamin D dogs need is approximately 225 IU per pound of food consumed, or 3.4 micrograms daily for an adult dog weighing 33 pounds and eating 1,000 calories.

- **Vitamin E.** This vitamin has an important role in the formation of cell membranes and in cell respiration. It is also a potent antioxidant that can help prevent the development of muscle disorders and cataracts. Dogs who get enough vitamin E usually have a glossy coat and healthy skin, but if there's a deficiency, problems with the fur and skin are among the first indicators. The recommended minimum daily intake of vitamin E is 2 to 20 IU.

- **Vitamin K.** Dogs make their own vitamin K, so there is no recommended daily dose. Normal blood function is synonymous with vitamin K: Without sufficient vitamin K, the blood does not clot properly. The main sources of vitamin K are egg yolk and green, leafy vegetables. Dogs rarely experience a vitamin K deficiency.

Minerals

A total of twelve minerals are essential for dogs, according to the AAFCO. They include calcium, phosphorus, magnesium, potassium, sodium, chloride, iron, copper, iodine, manganese, selenium, and zinc. Your dog's diet should provide all of these essential minerals in the right amounts and proper ratios, although it's not necessary that every meal meet these requirements. (A list of the minimum amounts of minerals required by the AAFCO in commercial dog food is provided in chapter 2, "Is Dog Food Fit for Your Dog?" where commercial dog food is discussed.) It's possible for dogs to get too much as well as too little of any number of minerals in their diet, so it's important to know what the recommended daily amounts should be. However, if you feed your dog a balanced diet using quality ingredients, you should not encounter any problems with minerals.

- **Calcium** is critical for strong bones and teeth, nerve impulse transmission, muscle contractions, and blood coagulation. Calcium deficiency can cause a condition called secondary hyperparathyroidism, which can occur in dogs whose diet consists primarily of meat. Signs include bone loss, bone abnormalities, and fractures. Too much calcium also can cause skeletal problems, especially in developing large-breed puppies. The calcium-to-phosphorus ratio is an important relationship to know when it comes to feeding your dog. For adult dogs, the ratio is about 1.2 parts of calcium for each 1 part of phosphorus (1.2:1), while the ratio is closer to 1:1 for puppies.

    Calcium can be challenging to provide for your

dog because it is not always easily digested and all dogs don't absorb it well. That's why it's common to see calcium as a supplement in homemade dog food recipes and why it is recommended for dogs who eat commercial dog foods. The amount of calcium for males and nonreproducing females is about 0.75 grams for a 33-pound adult eating 1,000 calories per day.

- **Phosphorus** works with calcium to support strong bones and teeth. It also plays a role in DNA and RNA structure, energy metabolism, maintaining the acid-base balance, and skeletal structure. The amount of phosphorus for males and nonreproducing females is about 0.70 grams for a 33-pound adult eating 1,000 calories per day.
- **Magnesium** has a role in bones and teeth as well, but is also essential to the integrity of muscle and nerve cell membrane health, the secretion and function of hormones, and the functioning of enzymes.
- **Potassium** is important for the proper function of nerves, muscles, and enzymes, and in keeping the fluid in your dog's body in balance. Potassium is found in many foods, so it's unusual for dogs to have a deficiency of this mineral. However, dogs who experience chronic diarrhea and/or vomiting or who have kidney disease or other conditions that deplete the potassium from their body may have a potassium deficiency. Symptoms of potassium deficiency include nervous disorders, loss of appetite, poor growth, weakness, and cardiac arrest. Excessive amounts of potassium are seen in dogs who have Addison's disease or hypoadrenocorticism, in which the adrenal glands fail to make enough of the hormone that regulates the amount of potassium in the blood.
- **Sodium** is necessary to help maintain proper fluid balance throughout the body, to transfer nutrients,

and to facilitate the elimination of waste from cells. Generally, sodium and chloride work together and are considered a pair, because they combine to make up table salt. Sodium is available in nearly every food to some degree, and therefore a deficiency of sodium is extremely rare.

- **Chloride** performs a variety of functions for dogs, including the production of hydrochloric acid in the stomach, which aids in digestion. Mostly chloride works with sodium to form table salt. A chloride deficiency is extremely rare because it is found in most foods, although dogs that experience severe diarrhea and/or chronic vomiting may have low levels of chloride.
- **Iron** is found in most meats, so an iron deficiency is uncommon unless you feed your dog a diet that consists mostly of vegetables and don't provide an iron supplement. Red blood cells require iron to transport oxygen throughout the body.
- **Copper** is necessary in very small amounts in dogs, but it is still critical for proper formation of cells, normal hair pigmentation, and the development of connective tissue. This mineral is commonly found in meats, so dogs fed a vegetarian diet may experience a copper deficiency unless they are given a supplement that contains the mineral and/or they are given grains that are high in copper. The copper in supplements should be in the form of copper lysine or cuprous oxide.
- **Iodine** is an important mineral because it is a major component of the thyroid hormone, and so most of the iodine in your dog is in his thyroid. The role of iodine in dogs is to assist with growth in puppies and with metabolism in adult dogs. Iodine is added to commercial dog foods, and it should be in the form of potassium iodide or calcium iodate.

- **Manganese** has a critical role in nerve function and bone development, and it also is involved in the overall health of the gums, teeth, and digestive system. Your dog can get manganese in her poultry, cereal grains, and seafood. Manganese as a supplement should be in the form of manganese carbonate.
- **Selenium** in your dog is found mainly in her muscles. Among the most important functions of selenium are as an antioxidant to fight infections and to support the immune system. Selenium is typically added to dog foods, and as a supplement, look for sodium selenate decahydrate or sodium selenite.
- **Zinc** is good for your dog because it is necessary for metabolism of protein and to help wounds heal, among other functions. The best food sources of zinc include red meat, whole grains, and peas. Zinc provided in supplements should be in the form of zinc sulfate, zinc oxide, or zinc carbonate.

   Zinc deficiencies are not common, but when they occur they affect the skin and fur. Certain dogs, including Siberian huskies and Alaskan malamutes, may have a genetic inability to absorb enough zinc, which means these dogs may need a zinc supplement to prevent a zinc deficiency and associated skin problems. In addition, if you feed your dog a diet high in fiber and/or plant foods or high calcium, your dog may develop a zinc deficiency. The recommended daily minimum for puppies and adult dogs is 120 mg/kg of food consumed.

SUPPLEMENTS FOR DOGS

It's been estimated that as many as one-third of dogs and cats in the United States are given vitamins or other supplements.

Leading the list are multivitamins, supplements for arthritis, and fatty acids. There is also a growing trend to give dogs supplements such as antioxidants that can fight aging, as well as probiotics (beneficial bacteria) to help manage gastrointestinal symptoms.

Why Dogs Need Supplements

There are several reasons dogs need supplements. If you feed your dog commercial dog food that says it is "nutritionally complete," your dog is getting all the essential nutrients she needs, right? More than likely, no. Even if you feed your dog a very high-quality commercial dog food, there is still a chance it is not providing everything your dog needs to stay healthy. The truth is, many people feed their dogs food that is of lower quality because it is less expensive and because they've been led to believe it contains all the right nutrients. And as you will learn in chapter 3, "What's for Dinner? Good Food for Your Dog," it is typically necessary to add one or more supplements to homemade dog food as well. After all, people take supplements, too, so why shouldn't your dog?

Many veterinarians recommend vitamin supplements for puppies to make sure they receive everything they need during their critical growth and development stage. Puppies are especially susceptible to getting worms (see chapter 17, "Worms [Intestinal Parasites]"), and a worm infestation can take a nutritional toll on young dogs, so supplementation can even be lifesaving for some puppies.

Aging dogs are more likely than their younger peers to experience health problems that impact the immune system, making it less able to fight off free radicals and toxins that cause disease. Older dogs are also less able to absorb nutrients from their food, and some of them tend to eat less. Therefore supplementation with various nutrients can be especially beneficial for senior dogs.

Finally, supplements—whether they are vitamins, minerals, herbs, enzymes, or other natural substances—can be helpful in managing a wide range of health challenges that your dog can face. You'll learn more about supplements used as home remedies in the chapters on dog conditions.

Do Supplements for Dogs Work?

Although there has been much research into the use of vitamins, minerals, and other supplements for people, the same can't be said about supplements for dogs. However, some supplements often given to dogs, such as glucosamine and/or chondroitin (for arthritis; see chapter 5, "Atopic Dermatitis"), some antioxidants, and omega-3 fatty acids have received attention from the scientific community. Unfortunately, when it comes to a popular doggie supplement—multivitamins and/or multiminerals—studies of effectiveness and long-term safety are in short supply.

As with supplements for people, there is always the question of whether the product actually contains what is advertised on the label. The Food and Drug Administration oversees supplements for pets, but another organization, the National Animal Supplement Council, has the task of establishing labeling guidelines and testing supplements for pets to make sure they contain what they claim on their labels. This nonprofit trade organization is made up of companies "committed to providing health supplements and nutritional supplements of the highest quality for companion animals, primarily dogs, cats and horses," according to their Web site.

You may ask, "Aren't nutritional supplements for my dog the same as the ones I'd take for myself?" and the answer is no. (However, herbal remedies for people are often used for dogs; see the introductory section to part II, "Canine Conditions and Home Remedies") Nutritional supplements for pets are typically formulated in ways that are specific for the animal, so it is best to use supplements that have been formulated for dogs. When they are not available, talk to your veterinarian about which human supplement is best.

How to Buy Dog Supplements

As your dog's health advocate and a consumer, you also have a way to check on the ingredients in some pet supplements: ConsumerLab.com, an independent group that tests nutritional products and issues reports for the public. ConsumerLab .com has a Web site you can access for further information. Generally, however, here are some guidelines for choosing quality supplements for your dog.

- **Look for products made by companies that have commissioned clinical studies of their supplements.** One way to discover if such studies exist is to visit the company's Web site and look for articles and research on their Web pages. Another way is to search PubMed (www.ncbi.nlm.nih.gov/pubmed/) and type in the search box the name of the supplement and/or the company to discover if any studies have been published.
- **Be familiar with the ingredients you want for your dog.** For example, there are many types of calcium; which one is the best for your dog? (Hint: Check out the section on "Calcium.")
- **If a supplement says it will prevent disease, steer clear.** Such promises are too good to be true
- **Select well-respected supplement makers.** These can include those offered by your veterinarian as well as others that have gotten good reports by Con sumerLab.com.
- **Look for products that list a lot number (which indicates the company has quality control standards) and contact information.** Call the com-

pany and ask about their product, including whether any studies have been done on the product and are available. Look at their Web site.
- **Look on the label for certification from an independent organization that has verified the contents of the supplement.**

Some dog foods, especially those formulated as therapeutic or prescription canine foods, contain specific supplements for particular conditions. For example, there are dog foods that contain glucosamine and chondroitin for dogs who are suffering with symptoms of osteoarthritis. Others may contain the omega-3 fatty acid DHA (docosahexaenoic acid) to help with cognitive dysfunction syndrome (see chapter 6, "Cognitive Dysfunction Syndrome [Doggie Dementia]").

Here are some common nutritional supplements pet parents buy for their dogs to supplement their dogs' food. These supplements may be used as ingredients in homemade dog recipes or given as supplements at other times either in food or alone. Several of these supplements also can be used to manage certain health conditions, and in those cases they are discussed in their appropriate individual chapters.

Multivitamins/Minerals

A multivitamin/mineral supplement may be recommended if you are making homemade dog food (many recipes include this supplement as an ingredient) and especially if you are feeding your dog commercial dog foods. If you are feeding your dog a high-quality dog food that has extra vitamins and minerals or a food that has been prescribed by your veterinarian, check with your vet before giving your dog a multivitamin/mineral supplement.

A good-quality multivitamin/mineral supplement should contain at least the essential vitamins, including vitamin A, D, E, and the B-complex vitamins (thiamin, riboflavin, niacin, B_5, B_6, folic acid, biotin, B_{12}). All the nutrients should be in ratios and amounts that will support your dog's health.

The individual ingredients also should come from natural, quality sources. If the sources are not revealed on the label, you may want to contact the company by phone or e-mail, or check their Web site to get the information. Examples of quality sources include cod liver oil, brewer's yeast, wheat germ, and liver.

Follow the dosing instructions on the supplement bottle, which typically are given according to your dog's weight. For example, the instructions may ask you to give your dog ½ tablet per 10 pounds of body weight, or one tablet per 25 pounds of body weight.

Calcium

According to Claudia Kirk, DVM, PhD, DACVN, DACVIM, a professor of medicine and nutrition at the University of Tennessee College of Veterinary Medicine, "Calcium is probably the most common deficiency in a homemade diet that isn't professionally balanced." "Professionally balanced" means you have consulted with your veterinarian or canine nutritionist to be sure your homemade doggie recipes are providing all the nutrition your dog needs.

Dogs who don't get enough calcium are at risk of developing nutritional secondary hyperparathyroidism, a condition characterized by abnormal bone growth, soft bones, and even fractures in severe cases. The risk of such bone damage is especially critical in young dogs who eat an unbalanced homemade diet. However, if you improve the diet, you can avoid or correct the problem, so talk to your vet.

Commercial dog food makers add powdered bonemeal or calcium carbonate to their products to help make sure dogs get enough of this critical nutrient. Dogs who regularly eat raw bones likely get enough calcium. And if you choose, you can give your dog raw bones on a regular basis to up her calcium intake.

But the meat and fish in homemade dog food, while great sources of protein, are also high in phosphorus, which inhibits the absorption of the calcium in the total diet when the calcium-to-phosphorus ratio is not optimal, which is about 1.2:1. The amount of calcium added to commercial dog food is 1 percent to 1.2 percent on a dry-matter basis, and you can achieve a similar amount using 750 mg of calcium carbonate tablets (crushed) per 10 to 15 pounds of your dog's body weight per day. Calcium citrate and bone meal are other options.

If you decide to use calcium supplements, choose those that do not contain vitamin D, because chances are your dog is already getting enough of this vitamin, and supplementing with the vitamin may be toxic, as too much vitamin D can cause bone and muscle damage.

MAKE YOUR OWN CALCIUM SUPPLEMENT

Don't throw away those eggshells! Finely ground eggshells can be used as a calcium supplement.

- Rinse eggshells and dry them on a flat baking sheet, either in a low oven for 1–2 hours or in direct sunlight.
- Grind the eggshells in a clean blender, food processor, or coffee grinder.
- Sift through a very fine sieve and regrind any pieces left behind.
- One-half teaspoon of finely ground eggshells provides approximately 1,000 mg of elemental calcium.

B Complex

The B family of vitamins are typically found in a multivitamin supplement and include thiamine (B_1), riboflavin (B_2), niacin (B_3), pantothenic acid (B_5), vitamin B_6, folic acid, biotin, and vitamin B_{12}. However, if your veterinarian has suggested giving your dog a B-complex supplement, the typical dose for dogs is as follows, twice daily: small dogs, regular potency; medium dogs, high potency; and large dogs, high-potency stress formula.

Vitamin D

If you give your dog a multivitamin/mineral supplement, then vitamin D is likely already in the product. Whether the vitamin D is in the multivitamin supplement or you are giving your dog extra vitamin D in a separate supplement, you want to make sure it's the right kind. Although people can transform calciferol (D_2) into active vitamin D_3, dogs cannot. When choosing a vitamin D supplement for your dog, look for ones that contain cholecalciferol (D_3) and not calciferol (D_2). The minimum recommended dose of vitamin D is 5 IU per pound of body weight or 225 IU per pound of food fed.

Omega-3 Fatty Acid/Fish Oil Supplements

An omega-3 fatty acid or fish oil supplement (omega-3 fatty acids are mainly found in fish oil) is recommended for dogs regardless of whether they are eating a commercial dog food diet or one that is homemade. That's because omega-3 fatty acids are known as essential fatty acids, which means the body cannot manufacture them and so they must be obtained from the diet.

The two main omega-3 fatty acids that can benefit your dog are EPA (eicosapentaenoic acid) and DHA (docosahexaenoic acid), and both are found in cold-water fish such as tuna, herring, salmon, and mackerel. EPA and DHA work together to reduce inflammation, maintain brain health, and various other health-related benefits.

Omega-3 fatty acid supplements for dogs are available as regular fish oil, salmon oil, or cod liver oil supplements. It is best to use fish oil or salmon oil supplements, because cod liver oil supplements are typically high in vitamins A and D, which often are not necessary to provide as a supplement and can be toxic at high amounts.

Omega-3 fatty acids are also available in flaxseed oil, but the omega-3 in this form is called ALA, which dogs must first convert to EPA before the body can use it. Since only about 15 percent of ALA is converted to EPA, the best way for your dog to get her omega-3s is from fish oil.

The suggested dose of fish oil for dogs is 1,000 mg (containing a combination of 300 mg of EPA and DHA) per 30 pounds of body weight. Another way to figure dosage is to supplement around 1.75 grams of EPA per kilogram of food and 2.2 grams of DHA per kilogram of food. As an alternative, you can give your dog sardines instead of fish oil supplement: One small sardine provides 100 mg EPA/DHA. Amounts of omega-3 fatty acids given for specific health conditions differ from these maintenance levels and are explained in their appropriate chapters.

Fish oil is available as a liquid and in capsules: Pierce the end of a capsule with a pin and squeeze out the oil into your dog's food. If you give your dog an omega-3 supplement, you should also add a vitamin E supplement as a complement. A recommended dosage is 1 to 2 IUs per pound of body weight per day.

HOW MUCH FOOD DOES MY DOG NEED?

A common question from dog parents is: How much food should I give to my dog? You can follow the guidelines on the bag of kibble you just bought, but if the nutritional value of that food is questionable—and it could well be—then you can use another gauge to help determine how much food your dog needs. Besides, the recommendations by a dog food manufacturer are questionable, because it does not know your dog. How much food your dog needs depends on your dog's age, breed, metabolism, activity level, environmental conditions, and whether she is overweight, underweight, pregnant, or trying to maintain weight. Dog food makers may overstate or understate how much food to feed dogs depending on whether they want to sell more dog food or try to make their products look like a better deal than their competitors.

In addition, if you decide to try homemade foods—and we hope you do—then some general guidelines for how much to feed your dog can be helpful.

The guidelines are presented using two different calculation methods, weight of food and calories, so you can choose the one that works best for you. Keep in mind that the amount of food/calories your dog needs is highly individual and depends on her activity level, her stage of life, her age, her environment, and even her breed. If you keep a close eye on your dog's weight, energy level, and health, you can better gauge how much food she needs.

Weight-of-Food Method

For most dogs, the amount of food they receive each day should equal 2 percent to 3 percent of the dog's total body weight. Growing puppies need more, and elderly or very inactive dogs require less. To calculate how much food you should feed your dog using this method, follow this example:

- A 35-pound dog $\times$ 16 ounces = 560 ounces, which is the dog's total body weight in ounces
- 560 ounces $\times$ 0.02 (2 percent) = 11.2 ounces, which is the total daily minimum weight of food to feed to your dog

OR

- 560 ounces $\times$ 0.03 (3 percent) = 16.8 oz, or the total daily maximum weight of food to feed to your dog
- This translates into about ¾ to 1 pound of food daily.

Calorie Method

On average, dogs need about 25 calories per pound of body weight per day to maintain health. Keep in mind this is the *average* only, and there is a range from 15 to 40 calories per day.

For example, dogs who weigh less than 20 pounds usually need 40 calories per pound per day. So if your long-haired dachshund, Limo, weighs 15 pounds, then he needs 600 calories per day.

For dogs at the other end of the scale, those who weigh more than 100 pounds, the number of calories needed per day is about 15 per pound. Therefore, if Tiny the bullmastiff weighs in at 125 pounds, he needs about 1,875 calories per day.

Chapter 2

Is Dog Food Fit for Your Dog?

A nutritious diet is the foundation of your dog's overall health. As in humans, at least half—and probably more—of the diseases and other ailments that can affect your dog can be prevented if he consumes a wholesome, natural diet. This chapter tackles the big questions concerning your dog's food: What is in commercial dog food? Is commercial dog food safe? Which types of commercial dog foods are good for your dog? How do you decipher dog food labels?

Commercial dog food is big business today, but it wasn't always that way. Before World War II, people fed their dogs meat and other foods that they ate (yes, table scraps). However, around World War II, people began switching from the traditional meat and meat by-product diet to commercial dog foods as they became more available, convenient, and affordable. A pet parent's dream, right? Or a nightmare?

THE BUSINESS OF FEEDING FIDO

You cannot be absolutely certain about the quality of the dog food you buy from commercial pet food manufacturers. In fact, most commercial pet food contains "feed grade" ingredients that don't meet the same standards as foods you would eat. One important example is the meat in dog food. As you probably know, dogs need protein, and the higher the quality, the better. Animal protein is the main protein source for dogs, and in the pet food industry that meat may come with a "four-D" label that indicates where the meat came from: dead, dying, disabled, and diseased animals. Although dog food makers will deny the four Ds represent any of their meat sources, there are also claims by individuals and pet advocates that these cheap yet technically nutritionally complete meat sources are part of the dog food market.

Despite the apparent variety of dog foods on the market, most of them are made by one of the following three huge international companies, with the first two exceeding the third one by more than threefold in sales:

- **Mars Petcare US:** makers of Pedigree, Royal Canin, and Nutro, among others
- **Nestlé SA:** makers of Purina Dog Chow, Purina Puppy Chow, Purina One, Purina Veterinary Diets, Purina Pro Plan, Mighty Dog, Alpo, and Beneful, among others
- **Colgate-Palmolive Co.:** makers of Hill's Science Diet, Hill's Prescription Diet, and Hill's Science Plan.

Many commercial dog food brands provide poor nutrition because they use low-quality ingredients and because of processing (e.g., high heat) and long-term storage, both of which can damage or destroy vitamins and enzymes as well as turn fats rancid. Add to this scenario the addition of fillers, artificial colors, flavors, preservatives, and other chemicals, and you have a meal fit for no one, and no dog.

The good news is that there are many much smaller dog food makers who provide whole, natural, and/or organic high-quality products for your dog. You won't find most of these dog foods on your grocery store shelves or even in some pet stores, but with just a little effort you can find them on the Internet, in select pet stores, and through veterinary professionals (see the appendix for a resource list). Another food choice is homemade dog food, which is covered in chapter 3, "What's for Dinner? Good Food for Your Dog."

Dog Food Regulators

The Association of American Feed Control Officials (AAFCO) is a nonprofit, voluntary membership group consisting of local, state, and federal officials who are responsible for enforcing their state's laws regarding the safety of animal feed and drug remedies. Some of its voting members are from the Food and Drug Administration (FDA) and the U.S. Department of Agriculture. Although the AAFCO has no regulatory authority, it helps develop and implement laws, regulations, standards, and enforcement policies regarding animal feed. The AAFCO has established minimum levels of nutrients that provide a balanced and complete diet for pets (see "Nutritional Requirements of the AAFCO" on page 45).

AAFCO review of pet food is voluntary. Any dog food maker can state on the label that their product has been formulated to meet the nutritional standards that the AAFCO has set, but this does not mean the dog food was approved by the AAFCO or that it was tested in any way.

The FDA's regulation of pet food falls under the Food, Drug, and Cosmetic Act, which requires that all animals foods be safe to consume, produced under sanitary conditions, free of harmful ingredients, processed to ensure it does not contain viable microorganisms, and labeled truthfully. Many of the ingredients and additives in dog food are considered to be "generally regarded as safe," or GRAS, which does not mean they are safe.

In fact, a significant number of preservatives, flavorings, and colors regarded as GRAS have been found to cause health problems in lab animals, yet they can still be added to pet food (and some human foods as well). The FDA's Center for Veterinary Medicine can take action to change or ban the use of an ingredient or additive in dog and other pet foods if it is found to be dangerous.

On an even darker side of dog and other pet food safety, there is concern among some pet parents and others about the apparent disregard of the FDA's regulations. There are compliance policies, which might be likened to tax loopholes, that apparently allow FDA regulators and field representatives to skirt the laws when it comes to pet food. According to TruthAboutPetFood.com, dead, dying, disabled, and diseased animals (the "four Ds"), and even euthanized pets, can find their way into pet food. In addition, ingredients that have been contaminated with rodent, roach, and bird excrement are also used for pet food.

Obviously this is a highly contentious and complex subject and a topic about which pet parents should be aware. Individuals who want to explore this area further are encouraged to visit TruthAboutPetFood.com and the Dog Food Project (see the appendix for links) and to explore books on the topic, including those by Ann Martin and Marion Nestle (see "Suggested Readings"), all of which reveal investigated activities of the pet food industry that may prove shocking.

PROCESSING DOG FOOD

Processing has a significant impact on the quality of a dog food. Most pet parents are familiar with only three or four different forms in which dog food is available, yet dog food is produced in a variety of forms, including dry extruded (kibble, the most common), canned, soft moist, shelf-stable moist, baked, refrigerated, frozen, dehydrated, and raw.

Although the initial meat ingredients for a dog food may be high quality, much of the nutritional value is lost during the rendering process, which uses high heat to dry the ingredients and separate the fat from the protein and bone, yielding grease or tallow and protein meal: meat meal, poultry by-products meal, and so on. The process of rendering reduces protein value, while the extrusion process, which transforms food into kibble, destroys even more nutrients. In an attempt to make up for the lost nutritional value as well as give the food a longer shelf life, it can be sprayed with highly preserved animal fat and vitamins. Processed dog food can also lose more nutritional value during transportation and storage.

WHAT'S IN COMMERCIAL DOG FOOD?

If you have ever attempted to decipher the nutritional information provided to consumers about commercial dog foods, you may discover that you'll need to brush up on your math skills and dig out your detective hat to figure out exactly what is in the dog food you buy off the shelf. That's because there are many terms to decipher and math calculations to be made before you can identify what's really in your dog's bowl—and even then there's no guarantee you'll have the answers.

Reading Dog Food Labels

It's time to get out your magnifying glass. If you are used to reading the ingredient panels on food you buy for yourself and your family, then you already know words can be deceiving, and dog food labels are no exception.

Dog food labels must list the ingredients in decreasing order by weight (on a dry-weight basis) rather than by amount or volume, starting with the heaviest item. If you read a label and the first four ingredients are "beef, corn middlings, corn gluten, corn meal," you may think the dog food mainly contains beef. Beef, like chicken, turkey, fish, and lamb, are whole-food sources that consist of about 75 percent water and therefore are naturally heavy. However, this example of a dog food label actually represents a corn-based food that has some beef in it. That's because the dog food maker has divided the corn into three different ingredients so it could list beef first.

Tactics like these are common in the commercial dog food industry, and it takes a savvy pet parent to decipher the labels in the quest for a high-quality food. But this is only the beginning of the detective work; there are dozens of other ingredients you need to understand if you want to find a healthful food for your dog, ingredients that involve meat by-products, meat meals, grains, vegetables, cheap fillers, and chemicals.

Yes, most dog foods contain artificial colors, flavors, stabilizers, and preservatives (such as BHA and BHT), all of which must be approved by the FDA or be generally recognized as safe (GRAS). Pet food makers must list the preservatives they put in their products, but they do not always reveal preservatives in ingredients that are processed somewhere else and added to their products.

Your dog doesn't need these artificial additives, preservatives, and chemicals you can't pronounce in his food (see "Deciphering Dog Food Ingredients" on page 38). Instead, look for dog foods preserved with vitamin C (ascorbic acid), vitamin E (mixed tocopherols), or plant ingredients such as rosemary. These natural ingredients do not preserve dog food as long as the chemicals do, so make sure to check the expiration date on any dog food that contains natural preservatives.

If possible, also avoid foods that contain meat by-products, especially those with the ambiguous term "meat" rather than a specific source. "Meat meal" may also contain meat by-products and are best avoided as well.

(RE)CALLING DOG FOOD

Any pet parent of a dog in 2007 probably remembers the huge cat and dog food recall by Menu Foods in March 2007. The company switched wheat gluten suppliers and found a cheaper source from a broker who imported from Chinese suppliers. The end result was pet food made with wheat flour laced with melamine, which causes kidney damage and led to the death of many companion animals. Scores of pet food brands were recalled, including Alpo, Best Choice, Cadillac, Costco, Diamond Pet Foods, Doctors Foster and Smith, Iams, Mighty Dog, Ol' Roy, Royal Canin, and others. The recall was the largest ever of consumer products in the United States. It brought to the forefront some of the horrors of the pet food industry and was the topic of the book *Pet Food Politics: The Chihuahua in the Coal Mine* by renowned scientist Marion Nestle.

Pet food manufacturers who issue a recall of their products typically do so individually as well as via a press release with the FDA. As your dog's health advocate, keep your eyes and ears open for pet food recalls in the news.

Deciphering Dog Food Ingredients

Here is a short list of some of the ingredients you can find in commercial dog food products. Those in **boldface** especially should be avoided. See the Appendix for links to dog food ingredients analyses.

- **Animal digest.** A substance obtained from the breakdown of unspecified parts of unspecified animals, which means the four Ds can be included, as well as roadkill, euthanized animals from shelters, and others.

- **Animal fat.** A by-product of the tissues of animals obtained during meat processing. The source is not specified and the fat is not required to come from slaughtered animals, which means the rendered animals can come from any source, including four-D animal sources, animals euthanized at shelters, and roadkill. The same warnings apply to **poultry fat**.
- **Artificial colors and flavors.** The exact identify of these ingredients is a mystery to pet parents. Labels may say "added color" or "artificial and natural flavors" without naming the sources. They add no nutritional value and may be harmful to your dog's health. Common artificial colors are blue 2, red 40, yellow 5 and 6.
- Ascorbic acid. This is another name for vitamin C and can help with metabolism. Dogs are capable of producing their own vitamin C.
- **Beet pulp.** This dried residue from sugar beets provides fiber but is also high in sugar and should be avoided.
- **Blood meal.** Meal made from the animal blood exclusive of hair, urine, and other extraneous materials except what might be included unavoidably during manufacturing. Consumers have no way of knowing the origin of the blood and what hormones, medications, or other substances may have been in it.
- **BHA/BHT.** Butylated hydroxyanisole (BHA) and butylated hydroxytoluene (BHT) are preservatives used to prevent fats from turning rancid. Many countries have banned BHA and BHT, but not the United States. Research shows that high levels of BHA and BHT can promote or contribute to cancer,

kidney and liver damage, dry skin, and dental disease in animals.

- **Corn.** Corn is an inexpensive filler, a common allergen among dogs, and a food that can be hard on the digestive system.
- **Corn bran.** Corn bran is the outer coating of the corn kernel and a common filler that has minimal nutritional value.
- **Corn gluten meal.** After removing most of the starch and germ from corn, what remains can be dried and made into corn gluten meal, which is a low-quality protein source. Corn gluten meal is a potential allergen for some dogs.
- **Corn syrup.** The concentrated juice extracted from corn. An unnecessary ingredient except that it makes your dog want the food more because of the sweetness.
- Dried whey. The substance that remains after removing water from whey, which is the watery part of milk. Dried whey contains not less than 11 percent protein nor less than 61 percent lactose.
- **Ethoxyquin.** A preservative that prevents fats from turning rancid. The FDA asked dog food manufacturers to reduce by 50 percent the maximum levels of ethoxyquin allowed in food after research showed the preservative might cause liver damage in dogs who consumed high levels. Ethoxyquin is also associated with reproductive problems, cancer, organ failure, and skin allergies.
- **Fish meal.** Clean, dried, and ground tissue of undecomposed whole fish or fish pieces. The fish oil may or may not have been removed. Fish meal is considered to be an excellent source of omega-3 fatty acids. However, any fish not destined for

human consumption must be conserved with ethoxyquin unless the manufacturer has a special permit.

- **Gelatin.** A colorless, nearly tasteless and odorless substance that is made by boiling bones, animal skin, and connective tissue. Gelatin is a binding agent used in dog food and also a source of protein.
- **Hulls.** This category includes oat, rice, peanut, and soybean hulls. Although a source of fiber, hulls are mostly a cheap filler with little to no nutritional value.
- Linoleic acid. An essential fatty acid (omega-6) found in most vegetable oils. Linoleic acid may appear on the label as soybean oil, lecithin, corn oil, linseed oil, or wheat germ oil.
- Meat. Meat is the clean flesh of slaughtered animals and can include the skeletal muscle, diaphragm, heart, esophagus, tongue, overlying fat, and part of the skin, nerves, sinew, and blood vessels normally in the flesh. However, the FDA does not allow pet food to contain body parts from animals who have tested positive for mad cow disease, nor can it include brains or spinal cords from older animals, who are at higher risk of the disease.
- Meat by-product. According to the AAFCO, meat by-products can include the blood, liver, brains, bone, udders, lungs, ligaments, stomach, and intestines. It is not supposed to contain beaks, hair, teeth, horns, or hooves, although some reports claim that it does.
- **Meat meal.** Rendered meal made from animal tissue. It is not supposed to contain blood, hair, hooves, horns, hide trimmings, stomach contents, or manure, although any of these substances that get into the meal unavoidably during processing are

allowed. Meat meal can contain up to 11 percent indigestible crude protein, which is protein your dog will not be able to digest.

- **Mill run.** Composed of the hulls of soybeans and/or wheat (may appear on label as "wheat middlings") and whatever sticks to the hulls. **Soybean mill run** and **wheat mill run** are often referred to as "floor sweepings" and are a cheap filler.
- **Natural flavors.** Flavor ingredients that are minimally processed and do not contain artificial or synthetic components. Their exact identity cannot be determined by the label, however.
- **Propylene glycol.** Used in antifreeze. In dog food, it helps keep semimoist kibble from drying out. Propylene glycol can be toxic if consumed in large amounts and is not an ingredient you want in your dog's food.
- Poultry by-product. Clean parts of slaughtered poultry, including the heart, lungs, liver, kidneys, feet, abdomen, intestines (free of feces or foreign matter), and head.
- **Poultry by-product meal.** This ingredient consists of the ground, rendered, and clean parts of slaughtered poultry, including the feet, neck, intestines, and undeveloped eggs. Feathers are not allowed except for those that may unavoidably enter during processing.
- **Rice gluten meal.** The dried remains after most of the starch and germ are removed from rice. Rice gluten meal is an alternative for dogs who are allergic to corn or wheat.
- **Soybean meal (de-hulled, solvent extracted).** Meal obtained by grinding the soybean flakes that remain after most of the oil has been removed from de-hulled soybeans using a solvent extraction process.

HOW TO MEASURE WHAT'S IN DOG FOOD

How much fat, protein, carbohydrates, and fiber are *really* in the food you feed your dog? I wish there were an easy way to answer that question, but unfortunately you need to do some calculations to arrive at an answer. There are three different ways to measure these nutritional items: by percentage of dry matter, by percentage of calories, and by grams per 1,000 calories consumed. Since the percentage of dry matter is the easiest and most frequently referred to in the literature—and the one usually used to figure out commercial foods—let's explain that one, beginning with the Guaranteed Analysis.

Guaranteed Analysis

On each dog food product label, manufacturers are legally required to provide a guaranteed analysis, which is the minimum levels of crude protein and crude fat and the maximum levels of crude fiber and moisture in pet food. ("Crude" refers to a method of testing the product, not to the quality of the nutrient.) Some dog food manufacturers also provide the percentage of other ingredients, such as calcium, phosphorus, sodium, and linoleic acid. You should note that the dog food may have more than the minimum or less than the maximum amounts stated on the label. One reason why exact amounts are not provided for these nutrients is that pet food manufacturers are always looking for the most cost-effective ingredients, so the quality of ingredients changes all the time.

Guarantees are given on an "as fed" basis, which means they are the amounts found in the dog food as delivered in the bag or can. This information is important if you want to compare two different types of dog food. Dry food (kibble) usually contains about 10 percent moisture, while canned, frozen, or fresh foods can contain 80 percent or more moisture. If a dog food label says a product contains 4 percent fat, you need to convert the "as fed" information into "dry matter," so get out your calculator to identify how much fat the food will give to your dog. To put it another way, you want to know how much fat is in the "dry matter," or the actual food minus the moisture.

Here's how to calculate dry matter when you have an "as fed" figure. Subtract the percentage of moisture from 100, then divide the "as fed" percentage by the amount of dry-matter percentage. For example, if you have a can of dog food that is 75 percent moisture:

$100 - 75 = 25$ *percent dry matter*
$4 \div 25 = 16$ *percent fat on a dry-matter basis*

Here's a shortcut: The amount of dry matter in dry dog food is about four times the amount in canned dog food. To compare guarantees between a dry and a canned dog food, multiple the guarantees for the canned food times 4.

You can use the same formula to calculate fat percentage for dry food.

If you want to know how many grams of protein are in a specific food, here's the formula. To convert the minimum percentage of crude protein into grams, multiple the crude percentage times the weight of the amount of food you give your dog daily. For example, if you feed Fluffy $\frac{1}{2}$ pound (226 grams) of food per day and the food consists of 8 percent crude protein, the grams of protein would be $0.08 \times 226 = 18$ grams.

If you are interested in the actual amount of total dietary fiber, you are probably out of luck, because if the label does not reveal soluble plus insoluble fiber as part of a complete nutritional analysis, there is no way to calculate the fiber content.

If you want to know the percentage of carbohydrates in a

commercial dog food, most manufacturers don't reveal that information. You can do your own calculations, however, by subtracting the percentages of protein, fat, moisture, crude fiber, and ash from 100.

For homemade dog foods, you can use the "percentage of calories" approach. To identify the calorie content of a recipe, look up each ingredient in the recipe in a nutritional calculator, such as NutritionData.com, and get the total calories and information on number of calories from protein, carbohydrates, and fat for each ingredient used in the recipe.

NUTRITIONAL REQUIREMENTS OF THE AAFCO

Here are the nutritional requirements for adult maintenance for pet food as established by the AAFCO. All the values are minimum requirements unless stated otherwise:

Protein . . . . 18 percent
Fat . . . . 5 percent
Calcium . . . . 0.6 percent (maximum 2.5 percent)
Phosphorus . . . . 0.5 percent (maximum 1.6 percent)
Potassium . . . . 0.6 percent
Sodium . . . . 0.06 percent
Chloride . . . . 0.09 percent
Magnesium . . . . 0.04 percent (max. 0.3 percent)
Iron . . . . 80 mg/kg (maximum 3,000 mg/kg)
Copper . . . . 7.3 mg/kg (maximum 250 mg/kg)
Manganese . . . . 5 mg/kg
Zinc . . . . 120 mg/kg (maximum 1000 mg/kg)
Iodine . . . . 1.5 mg/kg (maximum 50 mg/kg)
Selenium . . . . 0.11 mg/kg (maximum 2 mg/kg)
Vitamin A . . . . 5,000 IU/kg (maximum 250,000 IU/kg)
Vitamin D . . . . 500 IU/kg (maximum 5,000 IU/kg)
Vitamin E . . . . 50 IU/kg (maximum 1,000 IU/kg)
Thiamin (B_1) . . . . 1 mg/kg

Riboflavin (B_2) .... 2.2 mg/kg
Pantothenic acid (B_5) .... 10 mg/kg
Niacin (B_3) .... 11.4 mg/kg
Pyridoxine (B_6) .... 1 mg/kg
Folic acid .... 0.18 mg/kg
Vitamin B_{12} .... 0.022 mg/kg
Choline .... 1,200 mg/kg

All these nutrients are listed on a dry-matter basis, which means if you are comparing nutrient content in different dog foods, you need to take the moisture content into consideration. For example, a dog food that contains 80 percent moisture consists of 20 percent other nutrients. To determine how a specific nutrient in the food compares with the AAFCO recommendations, take a nutrient amount and divide by 0.20 to get the dry matter amount to compare. If the moisture content is 10 percent, then the rest of the nutrients make up 90 percent, so divide each nutrient value by 0.9 to get the dry-matter amount. Given the wide range between minimum and maximum for many of the nutrients, some experts and pet parents argue that the figures are virtually meaningless.

Chapter 3

What's for Dinner? Good Food for Your Dog

What's for dinner? Isn't that what your dog is asking when she waits patiently (or not so patiently!) with her tail wagging as you fill her bowl? Wouldn't it be satisfying if you knew exactly what you were putting in her bowl day after day?

In this chapter, the focus is on the basic tools you can use to provide your dog the most nutritious, health-sustaining, disease-preventing food possible, and in ways that are convenient and cost-effective. If you have children, ask them to help prepare homemade foods for your dog. This is a great way to get them involved in caring for your dog and learning about her nutritional needs.

Generally, the optimal diet for your dog is one that is based on whole, natural ingredients that provide a balance of protein, fats, carbohydrates, and nutrients that support and maintain your dog's physical and mental health. If this sounds familiar, you're right: The ideal diet for you and your dog are not so different.

This means you can do your health a favor by motoring past the drive-up window of fast-food burger joints, and you can do the same healthful move for your dog by trotting past most of the commercial dog foods on the market. Since you are her eyes, ears, wallet, and ultimate food provider, the choice is up to you.

You'll soon see that you can take what you've learned in the previous two chapters and create healthful homemade meals for your dog. Even if you choose to supplement a natural, high-quality commercial dog food with homemade fare rather than go 100 percent with freshly made food, you can still make a significant improvement in your dog's basic health. Once you try a few basic recipes, you'll see how easy and satisfying it can be to provide your dog with a home-cooked meal!

I don't want to leave you with the impression that there are absolutely NO worthwhile commercial dog foods on the market. For pet parents who would like to prepare home-made food but simply don't have the time and/or the inclination, there is an explanation and list of high-quality dog foods presented at the end of this chapter.

HOMEMADE DOG FOOD, GOOD AND EASY

A simple, well-balanced homemade diet can have an incredible impact on your dog's health. Why? Because the vast majority of commercial dog foods are made with poor-quality ingredients and contain added artificial colors, flavors, preservatives, and other chemicals that all together not only don't provide needed nutrition but can also cause allergic reactions and contribute to the development of scores of health problems. In other words, if you feed your dog toxic food, you lay the foundation for illness and disease.

If, however, you switch to wholesome homemade dog food (or a balance of high-quality commercial dog food and homemade fare), then your dog will have a stronger immune system and a better quality of life. A high-quality diet helps dogs avoid or reduce the burden of the common doggie ailments ranging from dental problems to fleas, allergies, diarrhea, urinary tract infections, and worms. Or, if they are affected by health problems, having a strong immune system will enable them to fight off the worst of the illness or disease and experience milder symptoms.

Commercial dog foods typically contain more than 50 percent carbohydrates that are difficult to digest (e.g., corn and corn meal) and contribute to inflammation throughout the body. Although dogs do need and enjoy carbohydrates and the nutrients and fiber they provide, the carbs should be high quality, not the cornmeal or corn by-products often added to dog foods.

Which Homemade Dog Food is Best?

The answer to this question is: That depends on you and your dog. There is no one "right" diet. Chances are, you don't eat the exact same thing every day. Nor should your dog. You like variety; so does your dog. When it comes to homemade dog food, there are different types of diets, including raw, cooked, a combination of raw and cooked, those that contain some grains, those that severely limit or eliminate grains, those that include dietary supplements, and those that combine some homemade foods with high-quality commercial brands.

If the idea of making homemade dog food is beginning to sound complicated, it's really not. Think of it like experimenting with your own diet. Some foods don't agree with you; that is, you have difficulty digesting them, or you are allergic to or intolerant of them. Your dog is the same way: Some foods, such as grains, may cause allergic reactions like itching and scratching (see chapter 5, "Atopic Dermatitis") or stomach upset. Then you will know to limit or avoid these ingredients in her food. With a minimum amount of effort, you can create homemade food your dog can eat all the time or as a complement to high-quality commercial foods. If you prepare a big batch each time and freeze individual portions, you will have a ready supply that lasts for days, even weeks.

When you make your own dog food, you have the advantage of knowing where the ingredients come from and how they are prepared. You can avoid processed, refined ingredients and adjust the components of each recipe as needed, based on your dog's weight, level of exercise, health conditions, and other factors. You can add and eliminate ingredients depending on how your dog reacts to them. You are in control.

Are all homemade dog foods healthy and nutritious? No, not if you don't use fresh, wholesome ingredients that provide the nutrients your dog needs. "Homemade" is not synonymous with "nutritious," just as "natural" does not automatically mean something is safe or good. (After all, dog poop is natural, but you wouldn't say it's good for you.)

A Vegetarian Dog Diet

Do real dogs eat vegetables? Sure they do! Although dogs are classified as carnivores, their metabolism is geared for an omnivorous diet. Therefore, they can meet their nutritional requirements on a vegetarian diet as long as it contains sufficient protein and is supplemented with vitamin D.

Many of the foods suggested for a vegetarian/vegan dog food diet are in the "Homemade Dog Food Shopping List" (see page 53)—all you have to do is ignore the animal products. Rather than meat, fish, and fowl for protein, the Vegan Dog Nutrition Association recommends legumes (e.g., pinto beans, soybeans, lentils, split peas, and chickpeas), which should be well cooked and either mashed or pureed. Other protein options include tofu, tempeh, texturized vegetable protein (TVP), and hummus.

The rest of the diet can include well-cooked whole grains (unless your dog cannot tolerate grains; quinoa, millet, oats, barley, and buckwheat are good choices), brown rice, sweet potatoes, cooked vegetables, and chopped raw leafy greens (e.g., spinach and mustard greens). Small amounts of fruit are also good, especially for snacks. A vegan dog food diet does not include eggs (an especially good protein source) or dairy products, so this approach is more restrictive than vegetarian fare, which can include the latter foods.

Two amino acids found in animal flesh but not in plants are taurine and L-carnitine. If you feed your dog a vegetarian or vegan diet, you will need to supplement these protein builders. Vitamin B_{12} is another nutrient you will need to supplement, since it is found in animal products. Commercial vegetarian/vegan dog foods should include these three nutrients, and you also can buy supplements that contain all three. Consult your veterinarian or canine nutritionist about the best supplements for your vegetarian/vegan dog. (See the appendix for some supplement sources, including those for vegetarian dogs.)

Raw Versus Cooked

The debate over whether a raw food diet is healthier or more nutritious than a cooked homemade diet, or whether it is even safe, is ongoing. Unfortunately, few scientific studies have examined the questions that revolve around this issue. A review of the scientific literature on the subject ("Raw Food Diets in Companion Animals: A Critical Review") was published in January 2011 in the *Canadian Veterinary Journal*, and the authors' conclusion was that "there is some compelling evidence suggesting that raw food diets may be a theoretical risk nutritionally" and that "raw food poses a substantial risk of infectious disease to the pet, the pet's environment, and the humans in the household." They also noted that "although there is a lack of large cohort studies to evaluate risk or benefit of raw meat diets fed to pets, there is enough evidence to compel veterinarians to discuss human health implications of these diets with owners."

That said, some experts say the best food for your dog is raw organic meats, perhaps with added vegetables. If you do choose a raw diet, then organic meats are recommended as a hedge against some of the possible problems associated with raw foods. If you are thinking about a raw food diet for your dog, consider these factors:

- **Cost.** Organic meats are not inexpensive and not always readily available.

- **Handling.** Some people are opposed to handling raw meat or are not comfortable doing so.
- **Digestion.** Some dogs have difficulty digesting raw meats and experience gastrointestinal problems such as vomiting, diarrhea, and loose stools when on a raw diet.
- **Parasites.** Raw meat can contain parasites in the form of eggs and larvae, which are destroyed when meats are cooked properly. These parasites can infect your dog. Some parasites can be eliminated if you freeze the meat first, but freezing will not get rid of all parasites.
- **Bacteria.** You don't need to look far to see the news reports about bacterial contamination of meats, fowl, and dairy products. The biggest culprits are salmonella and E. coli, both of which can be deadly.
- **Human contamination.** Dogs who consume bacteria can pass the organisms into the environment, where they can infect people. There is also the possibility of contaminating your own food if you handle raw meats and do not properly wash your hands, utensils, and dishes.
- **Incomplete nutrition.** Some experts argue that a raw meat and bones diet does not provide all the nutrients dogs need as stated by AAFCO standards. Others say dogs have a gastrointestinal tract and dental structure that have stayed the same throughout their evolutionary history, and so a raw diet is perfect for them. The debate over whether a raw diet is nutritionally complete or not continues.

So, raw or cooked? The bottom line is: Consider the risks and benefits, consult an expert, and then decide what works best for you and your dog. Veterinarians and canine nutrition experts everywhere report that well-planned cooked homemade foods for dogs are nutritious and support canine health. Preparing homemade food for your dog can be as easy or as difficult as you make it. We definitely want to make it as easy as possible, and so let's start with a homemade dog food shopping list.

HOMEMADE DOG FOOD SHOPPING LIST

Does the current shopping list for your dog say "1 bag Brand X dog food" or "10 cans of Brand Y dog food"? Well, it's time to make a change, and the new shopping list may look something like the one for you and your family, because your dog *is* a member of your family.

First we'll look at individual food items that can be included in homemade dog food. Naturally, you may not use all of these foods and/or your dog may not like or be best suited for all of these options, depending on any health issues or preferences. What's great is that there are so many foods from which to choose!

We also present information about raw versus cooked and vegetarian doggie fare. Finally, we offer several simple recipes you can make for your dog, using the ingredients discussed.

Meats, Fish, and Fowl

Beef
If possible, choose grass-fed beef for your dog. Beef is a high-protein source that also provides B vitamins, iron, selenium, phosphorus, and zinc. Of the many forms in which beef is available, ground beef is the easiest to handle. Most grocery stores sell three or four grades of ground beef, which may come under a variety of names: ground round (90 percent lean, 10 percent fat), ground sirloin (85 percent lean, 15 percent fat), ground chuck (80 percent lean, 20 percent fat), and ground beef (73 percent lean, 27 percent fat). Regular

ground beef has the highest fat content, so look for beef with lower fat content. However, you can mix about two-thirds extra-lean ground beef with one-third ground chuck. If you have some leftover beef from your own meals, you can add it to your dog's food; just cut off the fat and gristle and grind it if possible.

Chicken
Both ground chicken and chicken pieces are good protein sources. Skinless chicken breast is about 1 percent fat, while ground chicken comes in at about 15 percent. You can grind your own chicken with a meat grinder; just remove the skin. Grinding your own chicken can be more cost-effective than buying it already ground, and you also have the option of grinding the bones, which will add calcium to the meat.

Turkey
Ground turkey is sold in three grades: 1 percent, 7 percent, and 15 percent fat. All three can be good for dogs, and you can choose the level of fat that fits your dog's needs. Whole turkey and turkey pieces are also good for your dog, and you should offer a mixture of both light and dark meat, along with organ meats, if you choose turkey.

Fish and Seafood
Wild caught cold-water fish, such as salmon, sardines, tuna, and mackerel, are excellent sources of protein and omega-3 fatty acids, which help the skin, fur, and immune system. When served with their bones, these fish also serve as an excellent source of calcium. However, because of the possibility of mercury and other heavy metal contamination, limit the amount of fish you feed your dog. Farm-raised fish also have contaminants, including antibiotics that are fed to the fish to help prevent disease. Organically raised fish are not readily available. Cooked versus raw fish is recommended. Shrimp and clams are low-fat, high-protein choices as well.

Liver

Liver for your dog is available both fresh from the grocery store and freeze-dried in many pet stores. You can even use liver to make treats for your dog. Liver provides excellent levels of vitamin A, B vitamins (e.g., thiamine, riboflavin, niacin, pantothenic acid, and folic acid), and vitamin K, as well as iron. However, don't overdo the amount of liver you give your dog. Liver is rich in vitamin A, and too much of this nutrient can be toxic to dogs. If you use liver, do not give your dog more than 1 gram of fresh liver per kilogram (2.2 pounds) of body weight per day. Raw liver is a potential source of parasites and bacteria.

Dairy Case

Eggs

Eggs provide the most easily digested form of protein for your dog, and the protein is also of a higher quality than that found in meat, fish, or poultry. The protein in cooked eggs is more easily utilized by your dog than that in raw eggs. A caution concerning raw egg whites is that they contain an enzyme called avidin, which reduces the absorption of the B vitamin biotin. Too little biotin can result in fur and skin problems. Therefore you can cause a biotin deficiency if you withhold the yolks from your dog, so it is best to give your dog cooked whole eggs.

If your dog has stomach upset, cooked eggs can provide an easily digested form of protein. In addition to protein, eggs are a great source of riboflavin, selenium, and the fat-soluble vitamins A, D, E, and K, which are good for your dog's coat and skin. Eggs are easy to prepare for your dog: Make up a batch of hard-boiled eggs and mash them with the shells still on for added calcium.

Are you worried about high cholesterol from eggs? Yes, dogs can have high cholesterol, but eggs fed in moderation—two to six per week, depending on the size of the dog—are considered a safe and nutritious addition to the diet. If you use a homemade recipe that contains eggs, alternate it with one without eggs.

Dairy Foods and Cheese

Dairy foods provide lots of protein and calcium, and the protein content is similar to that of meats. However, dairy foods from cows also contain lactose, a sugar that many adult dogs cannot digest properly. Dogs who are lactose intolerant suffer with gas and diarrhea because the lactose ferments in their intestinal tract. However, you can offer your dog two dairy products that are low in lactose: farmer cheese and dry cottage cheese. You can also buy low-fat or fat-free cottage cheese, freeze it, and then pour off the liquid that accumulates on top when it thaws. This liquid contains most of the lactose in the cottage cheese.

Yogurt

If you choose yogurt for your dog, pick only products that do not contain sugars, artificial sweeteners, or any type of fat or fat substitutes (e.g., Simplesse and Olestra). But do select yogurt that contains live bacteria, as they are beneficial for the gastrointestinal tract and support the immune system. Yogurt is also a good source of calcium.

Grains, Legumes, and Seeds

Flaxseed

Flaxseed, either the ground seeds or the oil, is a healthy addition to your dog's diet. Flaxseed can be considered either a food or supplement, since you will see ground flaxseed as an ingredient in homemade dog food recipes. The addition of flaxseed to your dog's diet provides several benefits:

- It is a great source of omega-3 fatty acids, which are good for her skin and coat.

- The omega-3 fatty acids in flaxseed may also help with allergies (see chapter 4, "Atopic Dermatitis").
- It provides a dietary source of fiber. If you use flaxseed oil, however, your dog won't get the benefits of the fiber.

If you use flaxseeds for your dog, grind them in a coffee grinder or food processor right before you use them, because the fat in these seeds can go rancid quickly. Store flaxseed and flaxseed oil in the refrigerator in an airtight dark container.

Legumes

Legumes—beans, lentils, and split peas—are often neglected when it comes time to make homemade dog food because pet parents are afraid their dogs will have gas. However, when rinsed adequately and consumed in moderate amounts, legumes can provide a significant nutritional boost to your dog's menu, especially if you are following a vegetarian diet. Legumes are a great source of protein and fiber, and they are low in fat. At the same time, they provide iron, phosphorus, folate, thiamine, magnesium, manganese, and molybdenum, which plays an important role in detoxifying the body of sulfites found in processed dog foods.

Rice

Although some dogs are intolerant of carbohydrates that come from various grains and seeds, rice is one such source that is usually well tolerated. In fact, veterinarians often suggest you feed rice to your dog whenever he has an upset stomach or needs to eat bland food for a while. Rice is a fair source of fiber and also contains some protein, iron, calcium, and phosphorus. Avoid the highly processed white-grain rice and go for the brown varieties, which have a higher content of fiber and nutrients.

Oatmeal

Cooked oatmeal is good occasionally when your dog needs some additional fiber, when he has constipation, or for a change of pace. However, too much can cause loose stools. For dogs who are allergic to wheat, oatmeal can be a safe alternative source of grain and soluble fiber. Although you and your dog may both enjoy oatmeal, be sure the oatmeal you give your dog is cooked and made without sugar or other flavorings.

Vegetarian Protein Sources

Your dog doesn't need to be a vegetarian/vegan to enjoy these foods, but they are important options for pet parents who choose this dietary approach. Tofu, tempeh (fermented soybeans), texturized vegetable protein (TVP), and hummus (made from chickpeas) are common plant-based protein choices for dogs. Two other high-protein sources are the grain amaranth and quinoa, a grainlike food. Both are gluten-free and so perfect for dogs who cannot tolerate wheat and other grains that contain gluten.

Wheat Products

Some dogs experience an allergic reaction to wheat products, but others have no problem. The easiest wheat food to prepare for your dog is whole wheat pasta, which can be found in many homemade recipes for dogs. Choose a size and shape your dog likes best; they do seem to have a preference for different shapes such as shells and twists. Spaghetti can be messy for dogs to eat unless you chop it up.

Vegetables and Fruits

Apples

If an apple a day keeps the doctor away, how about the veterinarian? Apples are a crunchy and nutritious food for your dog, and feel free to keep the skin on (although wash it thoroughly first). You may want to core the apple first, however, if you are concerned about the amygdalin in the apple seeds. Amygdalin is a form of cyanide, a poison, and although your dog would have to eat large quantities of apple seeds to experience any damage, better safe than sorry.

Apples are a good source of vitamins A and C as well as fiber. So cut up an apple for your dog and let him enjoy the treat. A few words of caution, however, are in order. Feed your dog apples in moderation, because too many can cause loose bowels. "Too many" depends on the size of your dog, so you be the judge. Also, apples contain sugar—albeit naturally occurring sugar—so too many apples may contribute to weight gain and should be fed in limited amounts to dogs who have diabetes.

Bell Peppers

Green and red bell peppers are excellent sources of vitamins A and C, and they add great taste and nutritional value to your dog's meals; just steam slightly. Slices of raw bell pepper are great treats as well.

Carrots

Most dogs greatly enjoy carrots, either raw or partially cooked. Remember: The firmer the carrots, the better it can help clean your dog's teeth and freshen her breath as well. Carrots are a good addition to your dog's homemade recipes.

Celery

Celery is often thought of as a diet food for people, and overweight dogs can get some extra fiber and nutrients without the extra calories if they chew on celery stalks. Many homemade dog food recipes include celery, which supplies vitamins C and K and the B vitamin folate.

Cruciferous Veggies
There are about a dozen cruciferous vegetables (so named because of a cross-like configuration during their growing process), but the three cruciferous veggies dogs seem to enjoy the most are broccoli, cabbage, and cauliflower. All three are good sources of vitamin C and fiber, but broccoli is by far the best source of sulforaphane, a cancer-fighting substance, although cauliflower provides some as well. Other nutrients offered by these cruciferous vegetables include beta-carotene, copper, iron, selenium, and zinc.

Cucumbers
Cucumbers are another vegetable often thought of as a "diet" food, and so use it for that advantage if your dog is carrying some excess pounds. Admittedly cucumbers are not nutritional dynamos, but they are a good source of vitamin K, superlow in calories, and an easy treat for your dog; just be sure to wash the peel thoroughly.

Green Beans
Green beans, either raw or cooked, are a good source of fiber, vitamins C and K, and manganese. For overweight or obese dogs, green beans can be a nutritious low-calorie, high-fiber food to replace some of their regular food. Dogs also enjoy raw or frozen green beans as a treat instead of dog biscuits.

Mushrooms
Mushrooms are a good source of vitamins A, B complex, C, and D, and some varieties have been credited with helping fight cancer. Some pet parents find that dried mushrooms make good dog treats, especially for overweight dogs.

Pumpkin
The addition of cooked fresh or pure canned pumpkin (but not the flavored kind you use to make pumpkin pie) can en-

hance the fiber, carbohydrate, and beta-carotene (and thus vitamin A) content of your dog's food. Pumpkin also has medicinal purposes, as you'll see in chapter 8.

Spinach

Spinach isn't just for Popeye; your dog can be a wonder, too, if he eats his spinach. Chock full of vitamins A, C, and K, with the minerals magnesium and folate for good measure, be sure to include some spinach in recipes that call for greens or vegetables. Steam or cook lightly.

Squash

Similar to pumpkin, lightly cooked squash is a nutritious ingredient in homemade recipes because it is a good source of beta-carotene and fiber. Squash is available year round, with winter squash varieties (e.g., acorn, Hubbard, and spaghetti) typically higher in carbohydrates than the summer squash (e.g., yellow, crookneck, scallop, and zucchini).

Sweet Peas

Most dogs enjoy sweet peas and have no problem digesting them, whether they are canned, fresh (cooked), or frozen. If canned, use unsalted varieties. Sweet peas are an excellent source of fiber.

Sweet Potatoes

Sweet potatoes are a wonderful source of beta-carotene, fiber, vitamin C, vitamin B_6, and manganese, and dogs love them. Make sure they are well cooked and mashed. You can cook the sweet potatoes with or without the peels, and chop the peels if you include them in a recipe. Too much sweet potato can give your dog diarrhea, so follow the amount given in recipes that include sweet potato.

Here's a tip for a healthy and inexpensive treat for your dog: dehydrated sweet potato slices. Dry sweet potato slices in a dehydrator and store them in an airtight jar. Use them whenever your dog deserves a treat and when training.

White Potatoes
Boiled or mashed white potatoes (not raw) are great for dogs, as they are good sources of fiber, potassium, manganese, vitamin B_6, and copper. Do not give your dog potatoes that are greenish or have sprouted, and always wash the peels thoroughly.

Miscellaneous

Brewer's Yeast
Brewer's yeast is what's left over during the production of alcohol, and is not the same as the yeast used to bake bread, which can make your dog ill. Most dogs like the taste of brewer's yeast, and that's a good thing, because it is a rich and convenient source of the B vitamins. Recipes for homemade dog food often call for brewer's yeast, but feel free to sprinkle a small amount on your dog's food anytime, because it is good for her coat and skin, and aids the metabolism of carbohydrates.

GARLIC: SAFE OR TOXIC?

Is garlic good for your dog, or is it toxic? You are likely to see information on both sides of this question, so here's the bottom line: Garlic can be very beneficial when used for certain conditions and in specific formulations, but too much can cause problems. First, the benefits:

Garlic contains a high level of alliin, a sulfur-containing compound, that combines with an enzyme called alliinase to form allicin, which has medicinal properties. Research indicates garlic has antimicrobial activity against bacteria, viruses, fungi, and worms, and can help boost the immune system. Studies in people show garlic may lower blood pressure and fight infections. Garlic oil can be used to treat ear mites and ear infections in dogs.

On the downside: Garlic is potent, so it's important to choose the correct garlic preparation for your dog. Studies in dogs comparing raw garlic powder, boiled garlic powder, and aged garlic powder showed that the latter was the form that did not cause any undesirable side effects. Therefore, when giving your dog garlic, look for an aged garlic extract. Do not use enteric-coated garlic products, because they can harm the intestinal tract. However, if you treat your dog for worms using garlic, fresh garlic is the optimal choice (see chapter 17, "Worms [Intestinal Parasites]").

The suggested dose of garlic for dogs is ½ capsule aged garlic extract daily for small dogs, up to 2 capsules (in divided doses) daily for large dogs.

SUPPLEMENTING HOMEMADE DOG FOOD

Even if you use only organic, natural ingredients to make homemade dog food, you will need to add a few nutrients, especially calcium, and perhaps a multivitamin/mineral (see chapter 1, "Basic Nutrition: What Your Dog Needs," for supplement information). Homemade dog food recipes that have been developed by veterinarians or canine nutritionists typically specify whether you should add a supplement. If you decide to create some of your own homemade dog food recipes, you may need to add supplements, depending on the ingredients you choose. Always consult your veterinarian or canine nutritionist to determine which, if any, supplements you should add to make your homemade dog food more nutritionally complete.

Adding these supplements is important for all dogs to ensure they get the essential nutrients and do not experience nutritional deficiencies. This is particularly important if your dog is a picky eater or is ill. Any dog who has been diagnosed with a specific vitamin or mineral deficiency also should be given supplements as prescribed by a veterinarian. Nutritional deficiencies can cause havoc to the immune system and lead to a multitude of health problems.

SIMPLE RULES OF HOMEMADE DOG FOOD

When preparing homemade dog food, there are three main rules to remember: Use quality ingredients, strive for overall balance, and make a variety of recipes. Then there are the "minor" rules concerning doubling and tripling recipes, storage, and serving suggestions. Let's start with the main rules.

Quality Ingredients

We can't stress enough the importance of using quality ingredients. Isn't that one of the main reasons you are making your own dog food and not using commercial brands? Refer to the list of different foods you can use in your recipes, the recipes in this chapter and in others throughout the book, and those you get from your veterinarian or canine nutritionist. You know what quality ingredients are: natural, whole foods, organic if possible. The foods to avoid giving to your dog are basically the same ones that also aren't good for your health: refined, processed foods, and that means fast food, fried foods, foods that contain artificial colors, flavors, and preservatives, and those containing sugars, unhealthy fats, and lots of sodium. Just think: You can learn to feed both yourself and your dog a better diet!

Overall Balance

The overall balance rule is simple: As Cathy Alinovi, DVM, explains, if you are going to feed your dog homemade food, "he should have 40–60% protein [by percentage of calories per day, with] the rest fruits, vegetables, with or without whole grains." If your dog is still growing, then he will need more calcium than people food usually provides. If your dog is not eating edible bones, you may need to add some calcium to the recipes as well. This balance of protein and other nutritious foods—incorporating the other two rules, naturally—should make your dog a happy, healthy camper.

Variety

Do you like to eat the exact same thing every day? Well, your dog doesn't, either. Feeding your dog a variety of foods is recommended for several reasons. One, he deserves not to get bored with his food! Two, variety allows you to make sure he gets all the nutrients he needs. It's a myth that you must make every meal your dog eats a completely balanced one. Are each of your meals nutritionally complete? I didn't think so! But over a course of the day or even a few days, you typically (hopefully!) get the nutrition you need because you probably eat a wide variety of foods from the different food groups at different meals. You can feed your dog in basically the same way.

Variety means just that: Try different meats (including small amounts of organ meats), fowl, and fish, based on what your dog likes and can tolerate. Also choose from a wide variety of vegetables, some fruits, and whole grains (if you choose to include them). Homemade dog food is not boring!

RECIPES FOR HOMEMADE DOG FOOD

Get out your apron, it's time to cook! The following recipes have been taken from various veterinarians and canine nutritionists, and some have been modified slightly from their original presentation just to show you how you can use a variety of ingredients to make delicious and nutritious meals for your dog. With minimal planning, you can incorporate preparation of your dog's meals into your lifestyle with little to no disruption. Your dog will appreciate your effort: His appreciation will be in the form of his better health, higher energy level, and tail wagging whenever you dish out the recipes. And remember, variety is important, so feed your dog different recipes and/or combine with a high-quality commercial dog food.

BONE BROTH

Raw beef, chicken, turkey, lamb bones with or without skin and/or meat

Place bones in a large pot or Crock-Pot. Cover the bones with just enough cold water (about 2 cups or water per 1 pound of bones) to submerge the bones and add 2 tablespoons of cider vinegar per 1 pound bones. Let stand for one hour.

Bring the mixture to a low boil, reduce heat and simmer for six to twelve hours for chicken bones or twelve to twenty-four hours for beef bones. You can also cook the bones in a Crock-Pot on low heat. The bones will be soft when touched with a fork. Skim any fat off the top once the broth has cooled. Strain the broth through a sieve lined with cheesecloth or paper towel or a colander. *Discard the bones; do not feed them to your dog.* You can store the broth in the refrigerator for up to three days or freeze it for several months. Use the broth as an addition to homemade dog food or as a treat thirty minutes before or one hour after a meal, as it can aid in digestion after a meal.

Courtesy: Dr. Cathy Alinovi and Susan Thixton

Down-to-Basics Homemade Dog Food

This is a very basic homemade dog food recipe that is really dozens of recipes, because it allows you to choose the ingredients that best suit your dog from three categories. Ask your veterinarian about which supplements are best added to your recipe(s).

$1/3$ cup cooked lean beef, chicken, or turkey, chopped
$1/3$ cup cooked sweet potato, lentils, millet, beans, white potatoes, or barley
$1/3$ cup lightly cooked peas, carrots, green beans, Brussel sprouts, broccoli, cauliflower, winter or summer squash

Combine the three ingredients. Will feed a 20-pound dog for one day. This recipe is easy to make in bigger batches and freeze. Supplement each day's serving(s) with a multivitamin/mineral, omega-3 fish oil supplement, and calcium.

Chicken or the Egg

5 lbs cooked chicken or turkey
9 hard-boiled eggs, including the shells
5 cups cooked brown rice, barley, or millet
1 cup cooked sliced carrots or cooked green beans

Makes about 16 to 17 cups of food, which will feed a 20-pound dog for sixteen to seventeen days. Supplement with an omega-3 fish oil supplement and multivitamin daily

Vegetarian Dog Delight

1 teaspoon olive oil
1 clove garlic, minced
1 medium zucchini, sliced or cubed
1 sweet potato, cubed
1 large bell pepper, sliced
1 medium eggplant, cubed
$1/2$ cup water
1–2 hard boiled eggs or $1/2$ cup cooked tempeh

Sauté the garlic in the oil, then add all the remaining ingredients except the eggs and simmer for twenty to thirty minutes or until all the vegetables are soft. Cool before serving to your dog. Serve with chopped hardboiled egg or tempeh, divided to match the number of servings appropriate for your size dog.

Chicken Noodle Roni Dog Food

This one is from Cathy Alinovi, DVM, and Susan Thixton, authors of *Dinner PAWSible: A Cookbook of Healthy Dog & Cat Meals*. You can make several days' supply of this recipe and keep it refrigerated. The recipe as stated here feeds one 30-pound dog for one day (divided into two meals) and provides 500 calories, 36 grams of protein, and 16 grams of fat.

$1/2$ cup cooked chicken, no skin or fat, ground or shredded
2 tbs cooked chicken liver, ground
1 cup cooked whole wheat pasta
$3/4$ cup steamed tomatoes, diced
$3/4$ cup steamed green peas
2 tsp cod liver oil
400 mg or $1/4$ tsp finely ground eggshell
$1/2$ cup bone broth (see page 66); optional

Combine the chicken and liver in a bowl and mix well. Add tomatoes, peas, oil, and calcium, and mix well. Add pasta and mix again. If you are using the broth, add at the end.

HIGH-QUALITY COMMERCIAL DOG FOOD

Although many of the commercial dog foods on the market are of poor and questionable quality, there are some manufacturers who produce high-quality dog food—dry, canned, refrigerated, and frozen—that contain all-natural, human-grade ingredients, along with high-quality vitamins and minerals and often prebiotics, probiotics, and digestive enzymes as well. These foods are also noted for what they do not contain: artificial colors, artificial flavors, preservatives, hormones, antibiotics, corn, wheat, soy, and poultry by-products.

Naturally, these dog foods are costly, but for pet parents who do not have the time nor inclination to make homemade food, or who want a premium option to homemade foods, these products are available either on the Internet or, in some cases, from pet food suppliers and grocery stores.

The following is a representative list of high-quality commercial dog foods. These names were taken from an unbiased dog food comparison Web site called DogFoodScoop.com. The list consists of nearly 100 dog food makers and is updated regularly. Those presented here are among the best as rated on this site. Manufacturers who offer organic products are marked with an (O), while those that offer vegetarian options are marked with a (V).

Artemis
Blue Buffalo (O)
Dog Whisperer (Cesar Millan) (O)
Eagle Pack (some O)
Freshpet (refrigerated and frozen foods)
Holistic Blend (O, V)
The Honest Kitchen (O, V)
Merrick Pet Care (some O)
Natural Balance (Dick Van Patten) (O, V)
Organix (O)
Party Animal (O)
Solid Gold

If you are interested in these or any other high-quality dog foods, I suggest you visit the manufacturers' Web sites and read about their products before making a purchase.

PART II

Canine Conditions and Home Remedies

Before you and your four-legged companion leap into this section, here is some information for you to chew on. These tidbits are offered to help you and your dog get the most benefit from these chapters.

#1: The health issues in the following chapters were chosen based on several criteria, namely: (1) They are among the most common disorders or conditions that affect dogs; (2) these conditions can easily be treated with home remedies such as nutritional supplements, dietary measures, and herbal remedies; (3) the selected remedies have shown some scientific and/or widespread anecdotal evidence that they may be beneficial; and (4) the remedies are readily available for consumers. The size and scope of this book limit the amount of useful information that can be covered in a comprehensive manner. Therefore, if you do not see a specific ailment or disease in this book, that does not mean it cannot be managed or treated with home remedies. Consult your veterinarian or get additional information from the appendix of this book on relevant organizations to contact and suggested readings.

#2: You should consult a professional veterinarian and get a diagnosis before you start home treatment. You probably know your dog very well, and as your dog's health advocate, it's important that you provide your vet with all the information you can about your dog's habits, behaviors, and history. The information you provide will be most helpful in the diagnostic process.

#3: When choosing food for recipes, nutritional supplements, or herbal remedies for your dog, consider these tips:

- **Get the supplement in a form your dog will take.** You and your dog don't want every dosing session to be a battle. Chewable tablets, powders, and liquids (including tinctures) that can be added to food are preferable to pills and capsules for many dogs.

- **Supplements should not interfere with any other treatments your dog may be receiving.** Also make sure you are not giving your dog anything that can interact negatively with other medications or supplements he or she may be taking.

- **Determine the safest and most effective dosage of the supplement.** This can be a challenge, because many recommended dosages for dogs are based on veterinarians' experiences, not on scientific or clinical studies, and each dog's needs are different. That's why you need to consult a professional before initiating home remedies.

- **Supplements should be cost-effective.** If not, you will be less likely to continue treatment as long as necessary. However, also keep in mind that the supplement may prevent or eliminate a symptom or disease, which in turn could prevent costly veterinary costs down the road. If a supplement or remedy is available in a pill or capsule and these forms are more inexpensive than liquid or powders, you should ask a professional whether you can crush the pills or open up the capsules to deliver the remedy to your dog.

- **Don't give your dog supplements or remedies designed for people unless you first ask your veterinarian's advice and you show him or her exactly which supplement or remedy you want to use.** Not only are dosages for dogs and people different, but supplements made for you might not taste good to your dog, they may contain extra ingredients that may harm your dog, and they could even be more expensive than getting a product specially made for dogs. That said, you can refer to "Herbal Doses for Dogs" on page 74 as a guideline and a point of discussion with your veterinarian if you choose to use "people herbs" to treat your dog.

#4: In any discussions about research studies, there are some terms you should know. "Randomized" means the study subjects were randomly assigned to their groups. A "controlled" study means there was a group in the study that did not receive the active ingredient. For example, ten dogs may be given vitamin C mixed in their food while the control group would be given food without the vitamin. "Double-blind" means neither the study's authors nor the vets and/or pet parents knew which dogs were getting the active ingredient in the study (e.g., the herb, supplement, or nutrient).

#5: Each chapter offers the top three to five effective and commonly used home remedies for each condition. If there are other supplements or remedies that may have some merit, they are listed separately under "Other Home Remedies You Might Try," with a brief explanation of each.

HERBAL DOSES FOR DOGS

A growing number of holistic veterinarians and pet parents are using herbal remedies for their dogs, yet finding herbal supplements specifically for dogs can be a challenge. Therefore, you will often need to turn to herbal remedies available for people and adjust the dosage. The following information on dosing with herbs for dogs are general guidelines only: Make sure you discuss with your veterinarian the most appropriate doses for your dog for each individual herb and/or condition for which you plan to give an herbal remedy.

Tablets. Tablets are usually not recommended for dogs. Use another form of the herb.

Capsules. Give one 500-mg capsule for each 25 pounds of your dog's weight, two to three times per day. Capsules typically can be opened and the contents added to food.

Tinctures. Give 5 to 10 drops for each 10 pounds of your dog's weight, two to three times daily.

Powder. Give $\frac{1}{2}$ to 1 teaspoon of powder for each 25 pounds of your dog's weight two to three times daily.

Fresh herbs/tea. The best way to give a dog fresh herbs may be in a tea that you add to her food. Use 4 grams of fresh herbs to make a strong tea: Allow the herbs to steep for fifteen to twenty minutes in 1 cup of boiled water, then allow the tea to cool before giving it to your dog, two to three times a day.

WARNING: Do not give any herbal remedy to a dog who is pregnant or lactating without first consulting your veterinarian.

Chapter 4

Arthritis

Does it take your pooch longer to get up from a reclining position than it used to? Is your four-legged companion less enthused about chasing a ball or going for walks? Does your dog fidget or seem to have trouble getting comfortable when lying down or sitting? Has your dog exhibited signs of lameness? These behavior changes could all be indications that your canine companion is suffering with arthritis, one of the most common health problems dogs share with their two-legged companions. (See "Signs of Arthritis in Dogs" on page 76.)

Arthritis is an inflammatory disease characterized by inflamed joints, swelling, stiffness, and pain. In dogs as in people, the two most common types of arthritis that develop are osteoarthritis and rheumatoid arthritis, with the former being far more prevalent. The joints most often affected in dogs are the hips, but the knees, shoulders, elbows, and ankles are also involved. A less common type of arthritis, called spondylosis, can occur in the joints between the vertebrae of the spine, but fortunately this form of arthritis rarely causes symptoms.

Arthritis in dogs is not a deadly disease, but some pet parents find themselves in a situation where arthritis has made it nearly impossible for their dog to stand or walk any longer. That's when they are faced with making the ultimate decision—the decision no pet parent ever wants to make. However, when arthritis is recognized and treated effectively—and this can be done without drugs—many dogs can enjoy a long and happier quality of life.

SIGNS OF ARTHRITIS IN DOGS

If your dog displays any of the following signs or symptoms for more than two weeks, a vet visit is in order:

- difficulty standing or sitting
- sleeping more
- movements that suggest stiff or sore joints
- increase in weight
- favoring a limb
- decline in activity level
- behavior or mood changes
- reluctance to run or climb stairs
- decline in alertness
- lameness.

WHICH DOGS GET ARTHRITIS?

Any dog can get arthritis, but in more than 75 percent of cases, the condition develops in dogs aged ten years and older. When it appears in younger dogs, it is often caused by hip dysplasia, a common disorder that affects the hip joint most often in larger breeds and breed mixes, such as Great Danes, mastiffs, German shepherds, Pyrenees, and similar breeds. (See "Arthritis and Canine Hip Dysplasia Are NOT the Same Thing" on the facing page.)

CAUSES OF ARTHRITIS IN DOGS

Approximately 20 percent of dogs develop osteoarthritis during their lifetimes. Arthritis can be caused by a number of factors, including hip dysplasia, ruptured cruciate ligaments (ligaments that surround the knee), a dislocated kneecap (a common problem in dogs), trauma to the joints, and other joint conditions. Being overweight or obese does not cause arthritis, but it typically places excessive strain on the joints and ligaments and makes the condition worse.

ARTHRITIS AND CANINE HIP DYSPLASIA ARE NOT THE SAME THING

It's a common mistake: Many people believe arthritis and canine hip dysplasia are the same condition, but they are not. **Canine hip dysplasia is a cause of arthritis.** Here are a few other things to know about canine hip dysplasia and arthritis:

- **Canine hip dysplasia is a malformation of the hip joint on one or both sides.** The malformation prevents the femur (the long bone in the leg) from fitting correctly into the pelvic socket, and it can also result in poorly develop muscles in the pelvic region.
- **Dogs can be born with canine hip dysplasia or develop it later.** In either case it can lead to the development of arthritis years later.
- **Canine hip dysplasia may also develop in puppies who are exercised excessively, who grow too rapidly, or who get injured.** This leads to hips that cannot develop properly.
- **Dogs with a poorly develop hip joint(s) typically compensate by moving differently in an effort to reduce pain.** As the body

(continued)

compensates, problems arise in other areas, including the spine, knees, and other joints.

- **Chronic compensation and misuse of the hip and other joints can lead to inflammation and arthritis.**

DIAGNOSING ARTHRITIS IN DOGS

If your dog is showing any of the signs of arthritis, it is important to get an accurate diagnosis before you begin treatment at home. Other conditions, including neurological disorders such as doggie dementia, cervical disease, and degenerative myelopathy (deterioration of nerves in the spine), can cause similar symptoms and need to be ruled out. Diagnosis of arthritis is usually made using X-rays, and arthritis will show as bone spurs where the ligaments and the joint capsule attach to the bone and by varying amounts of space and bone density around joints.

CONVENTIONAL TREATMENTS

Dogs and humans may both experience arthritis, but that doesn't mean they can share medications. That's not what we mean by home remedies! Although it's true that some of the medications you might take to treat arthritis belong to the same class of drugs prescribed for dogs, specific arthritis medications have been developed for pets, mainly because our four-legged companions have greater problems with toxicity.

In fact, use of arthritis medications for dogs can be risky, because little is known about the long-term side effects of chronic use (longer than one year) of these drugs. Because arthritis is a chronic condition, it is very possible your dog will need treatment for more than a year, and that is a factor you should consider when thinking about how to treat your arthritic dog.

Another consideration is that arthritis usually affects older dogs, who may already have other health issues, such as kidney, liver, or heart disease. How will use of arthritis medications impact these conditions? Is your dog already being treated for another disease? These are questions you will need to discuss with your veterinarian.

Let's consider the two main classes of drugs often prescribed for dogs who suffer with arthritis: nonsteroidal anti-inflammatory drugs (NSAIDs) and corticosteroids.

Nonsteroidal Anti-inflammatory Drugs (NSAIDs)

Nonsteroidal anti-inflammatory drugs work by inhibiting the activity of chemicals (prostaglandins) that cause inflammation and pain. These benefits are accompanied by potential side effects, including gastrointestinal bleeding, kidney disease, ulcers, liver disease, damage to articular cartilage (the cartilage that lines the joints), behavioral problems, immune disease, and even death. Therefore, it is important that your dog be examined before taking these drugs to determine if she has liver, heart, or kidney problems and whether it is safe for her to take these medications.

The more common NSAIDs prescribed for dogs for treatment of arthritis/osteoarthritis are (in alphabetical order): carprofen (Rimadyl, caplets, chewable tablets, injection, or generic form Novox as caplet), deracoxib (Deramaxx chewable tablet), etodolac (EtoGesic tablet), firocoxib (Previcox chewable tablet), and meloxicam (Metacam oral drop or injection).

General advice regarding the use of NSAIDs in dogs with arthritis comes from Shawn Messonnier, DVM, author of *The Natural Vet's Guide to Preventing and Treating Arthritis in Dogs and Cats*. Messonnier notes that "NSAIDs are best used at the lowest dose needed to maintain patient comfort, and only on an as-needed basis."

Corticosteroids

Corticosteroids also work by interfering with the activity of prostaglandins and so reduce inflammation and pain, but they are more potent than NSAIDs and the side effects can be more serious. Here's why corticosteroids can pose a problem for your dog:

Corticosteroids (steroids) are hormones that are produced by the adrenal glands. When you give a dog corticosteroids, his adrenal glands stop making the hormone. This work stoppage may not pose a significant problem if your dog takes a low dose of steroids for about a week to ten days. Short-term side effects may include an increase in appetite, an increase in water intake, and an increase in urination.

However, taking stronger steroids for a longer time places your dog at risk of infection because they suppress the immune system. Long-term use of corticosteroids in dogs may also result in destruction of the arthritic joints; metabolic problems such as diabetes and obesity; nervous system issues such as hyperactivity; vision problems; respiratory failure; skin problems; hair loss; high blood pressure; water retention; and gastrointestinal upset such as ulcers and pancreatitis.

In short, corticosteroids can play havoc with your dog's health, even though your purpose in giving them is to attempt to improve his quality of life. Corticosteroids that may be prescribed for your dog include hydrocortisone, prednisone, prednisolone (Solu-Delta-Cortef), dexamethasone (Azium), beta-methasone, and triamcinolone.

Messonnier, like many other vets who practice natural, integrative veterinary medicine, turns to supplements, herbal remedies, and other alternative methods to treat dogs with arthritis and relies on NSAIDS and other conventional medications on a limited basis, if at all. Your dog—and you—

have many choices when it comes to treating arthritis, and many of those choices include natural home remedies.

HOME REMEDIES

Many dog parents who use natural home remedies for treating arthritis are grateful these options are available, not only because they are effective and safe, but also because arthritis typically requires long-term care. While medicating your dog with harsh drugs can result in serious side effects that further destroy her articular cartilage as well as reduce her quality of life, natural remedies offer your companion a better chance to live well with arthritis.

That said, every dog is different, and no natural supplement or remedy will cure the disease. While nutritional and herbal supplements are not drugs, they can be potent (and you want them to be!), and so they should be used with care and forethought.

Diet

Foremost on the list of home remedies for arthritis is a nutritious diet that helps your dog maintain a healthy weight. If your dog has been eating according to the recommendations in part I of this book, that is a great start. If not, it's not too late to make some adjustments to your dog's menu. Homemade foods are best, and there are several recipes in chapter 3 ("What's for Dinner? Good Food for Your Dog") you can try. The second-best alternative is to feed your dog the most natural, minimally processed dog foods possible, with limited grains. Why?

Once a dog has arthritis, his body has difficulty with metabolizing calcium. While meats are generally low in calcium and high in phosphorus, grains are the opposite: higher in calcium and lower in phosphorus.

If your dog is overweight or obese, the time to help him lose excess pounds is NOW (see chapter 13, "Obesity"). An overweight or obese dog who also has arthritis will suffer (needlessly) more than a dog at optimal weight. Excess weight places too much stress on your dog's joints, worsens symptoms, and defeats your other efforts to provide relief. The loss of just 5 percent of a dog's weight—that's only 2.5 pounds for a 50-pound dog—can make a big difference in a dog who has arthritis.

Exercise

If you have arthritis and your joints are achy and creaky, you might not feel like exercising, but you know you should. The same goes for your dog, but it's critical that you don't overdo it. Let your dog set the pace: If she is reluctant to walk or slows down significantly partway through a walk, then it's time to stop. Excessive exercise can cause more damage to the joints.

Avoid long, pounding runs through the park. Moderate exercise is best: That includes walking and perhaps swimming if there is a pool or safe water source nearby. Swimming is excellent for arthritic dogs because it reduces stress on the joints. Regular exercise can also help with weight loss.

Omega-3 Fatty Acids

Omega-3 fatty acids can be added to the diet to help reduce inflammation. The two omega-3s that are best for dogs are eicosapentaenoic acid (EPA) and docosahexaenoic acid (DHA), both of which are derived from cold-water fish, such as tuna and salmon. You may be familiar with another omega-3, alpha-linolenic acid (ALA), which is found in flaxseed, walnuts, and green leafy vegetables. The body needs to convert ALA into EPA and DHA, but unfortunately, dogs (and cats) are unable to make this conversion. Therefore, omega-3 sources for your dog need to come from EPA and DHA.

It's important to realize that it takes time for omega-3s to become incorporated into the body's cells, so don't expect to see an improvement after just a month or so. However, if you add omega-3s to your dog's diet daily, these fatty acids will eventually help maintain healthier cells that resist inflammation.

Studies of Omega-3 Fatty Acids

Fortunately, arthritis is one of the conditions in dogs for which there are some scientific studies. One 2010 study conducted at the Kansas State University compared the effect of omega-3 fatty acid supplementation versus no supplement among dogs with osteoarthritis. Thirty-eight dogs were randomly assigned to receive either typical commercial food or food with added 3.5 percent omega-3 fatty acids as fish oil. All the dogs underwent orthopedic evaluations before, during, and after the ninety-day trial, and all the pet parents were questioned as well.

The dogs that consumed the omega-3 fatty acids showed significant improvements in several areas, including lameness and weight bearing, when compared with the control dogs.

Another study from the same university looked at the impact of both omega-3 and omega-6 fatty acids in dogs with osteoarthritis. The randomized, double-blind, controlled clinical trial included 127 dogs with osteoarthritis in at least one joint. The dogs were brought to one of the 18 veterinary clinics that participated in the study by their pet parents.

The dogs were randomly assigned to be fed a typical commercial food (control food) or a food that contained a 31-fold increase in omega-3 fatty acids and a 34-fold decrease in the omega-6 to omega-3 ratio compared with the control food. The study lasted six months, and both before and throughout the study the dogs were examined and blood samples were collected.

The researchers reported that the dogs who consumed the supplemented food had significantly higher concentrations of omega-3 fatty acids and significantly lower concentrations of arachidonic acid (an omega-6 fatty acid associated with inflammation and pain) throughout the study. Dogs who consumed the supplemented food had a significantly improved ability to get up from a resting position and to play at six weeks into the study, and an improved ability to walk at three and six months compared with the control dogs.

If your dog is taking prescription medication for arthritis, such as carprofen, use of omega-3 fatty acids could allow you to significantly reduce the drug dose, and may even let you stop it altogether (with your vet's approval, of course). A study published in the *Journal of the American Veterinary Medicine Association* reported on dogs with osteoarthritis who were taking carprofen and who were then randomly given omega-3 in their food. Over a three-month period, the veterinarians were able to significantly reduce the carprofen dosage markedly faster among dogs who were taking omega-3 than those who were not.

Omega-3 for Your Dog

As a point of reference, a suggested dose of omega-3 fatty acids for optimal anti-inflammatory benefit is 20 to 30 mg of EPA and DHA per pound of body weight, given twice daily. This dose represents the amount of EPA and DHA itself and not the amount of the oil. For example, if your dog weighs 50 pounds, then he or she would need to take 100 to 150 mg of EPA and DHA twice daily. If you have a 250-mg fish oil capsule that contains 150 mg of EPA and DHA, your dog would need to take one capsule twice a day. (Note: Prick the capsule with a pin and squeeze the oil into your dog's food.) Naturally, ask your vet for the optimal dose for your dog's needs.

Glucosamine and Chondroitin

Both glucosamine and chondroitin are considered chondro-protective agents, which means they help protect the cartilage as well as restore and repair it. Glucosamine and chondroitin also are excellent supplements to be used with omega-3 fatty acids. Let's look at each supplement separately first.

Glucosamine is a type of sugar that is found in various body tissues, including bone. This substance works in several ways to help with arthritis: It activates cartilage cells (chondrocytes), promotes production of other compounds important for healthy cartilage and joints (e.g., proteoglycans, glycosaminoglycans, collagen, and hyaluronic acid), and inhibits enzymes that can destroy cartilage. Studies in both pets and people show that glucosamine can be just as effective as NSAIDs in relieving arthritis symptoms—and without the side effects associated with NSAIDs.

Chondroitin also is a type of sugar and the main glycos-aminogylcan found in cartilage and joint tissue. Like glucos-amine, chondroitin stimulates chondrocytes to make cartilage and proteoglycans, boosts levels of hyaluronic acid, and appears to inhibit enzymes that can destroy the joints.

Glucosamine and Chondroitin for Your Dog

Glucosamine and chondroitin are often used together, and they are most effective when supplementation is started as soon as you notice symptoms, because these supplements act on living cartilage cells. Your veterinarian will likely recommend you start at a high dose for about four to eight weeks, after which time you can lower it. Generally, the suggested starting dose for glucosamine is 300 mg to 750 mg for a 20- to 40-pound dog and 1,000 mg to 2,000 mg for a heavier dog, one to two times daily. For chondroitin, the starting dose is 200 mg to 400 mg for small- and medium-sized dogs and 800 mg to 1,000 mg for heavier dogs. Glucosamine and chondroitin are also frequently used along with MSM. (See "MSM" below.)

Glucosamine is derived from shellfish, so if your dog has an allergy to shellfish, he or she should not take this supplement. Three different forms of glucosamine are available: glucosamine hydrochloride, glucosamine sulfate, and N-acetylglucosamine. The first two appear to be more effective than the latter form.

Glucosamine and Chondroitin Studies

A 2011 study published in the *Journal of Animal Physiology and Animal Nutrition* compared placebo with the use of collagen alone, glucosamine (2,000 mg) plus chondroitin (1,600 mg), and all three compounds together. The dogs were treated for 150 days and examined every month. Based on observations, the dogs in the three different treatment groups showed a significant reduction in pain.

In a 2007 *Veterinary Journal* study, thirty-five dogs with osteoarthritis were treated with either glucosamine and chondroitin or carprofen (control group). After seventy days of the study, the dogs treated with glucosamine and chondroitin showed significant improvements on scores for pain, severity of arthritis, and weight bearing. Dogs in the control group also improved, but they did so before the glucosamine/chondroitin group.

MSM

MSM (methylsulfonylmethane) is a potent antioxidant and a naturally occurring sulfur compound produced by plankton, but it is also found in meats, seaweed, cow's milk, fruits, and vegetables. The body stores sulfur in all cells of the body, but the highest concentrations are found in the joints, hair, and skin. Sulfur is necessary for the synthesis of connective tissue and cartilage, which is why MSM is helpful in treating arthritis.

Levels of MSM in the body naturally decline with age, and in dogs the reduction in the sulfur compound can show up as joint pain, arthritis, dull fur, and skin problems. Research suggests that the level of sulfur in arthritic cartilage is about one-third the amount in healthy cartilage.

Although studies of MSM and arthritis are mainly limited to humans, the results have been positive. Anecdotal reports from veterinarians on the use of MSM in dogs with arthritis are generally glowing as well. Use of MSM is associated with a significant reduction in inflammation, pain, and stiffness of joints, with an accompanying improvement in function and mobility. MSM is a facilitator, which means it helps nutrients move into cells while also pushing toxins out, allowing connective tissues to heal.

The optimum dosing and supplementation schedule for MSM will vary for each dog, but Dr. Messonnier recommends starting at 500 mg per 25 pounds of a dog's body weight, taken one to two times per day. Some experts recommend a lower dose, about 50 to 100 grams per 10 pounds of body weight. You may want to start low and gradually increase the dose. Side effects associated with use of MSM are rare, but occasionally it has been known to cause vomiting, diarrhea, and headache in humans. Infrequently, dogs given MSM have experienced changes in the lens of the eye, so you should have your dog's eyes checked if he is taking MSM.

MSM is available in tablets, liquid, and powder, and the latter two are easily added to a dog's food. Among the advantages of MSM are that it is tasteless, easy to use, and relatively inexpensive. It is common to use MSM along with glucosamine and chondroitin in dogs with arthritis, and supplements that combine the three ingredients are available.

Other Home Remedies

- **Dimethylglycine (DMG).** Dimethylglycine is formed naturally in the body when the amino acid glycine bonds with two methyl groups (a carbon atom plus three hydrogen atoms). Small amounts of DMG are found in meats, grains, and seeds. Research in animals (but not dogs) have indicated DMG may be helpful in relieving arthritis symptoms. Consult your veterinarian for the best dose for your dog.

- **Green-lipped mussel.** Also referred to as perna (*Perna canaliculus*), the green-lipped mussel reportedly provides some relief from arthritis symptoms in dogs based on the results of several studies, including one published in the *New Zealand Veterinary Journal*. However, for ecological reasons, use of green-lipped mussels is not recommended.
- **Vitamin C.** This potent antioxidant may help minimize or prevent arthritis in dogs if supplementation is started before arthritis develops. The form of vitamin C believed to provide the best results for dogs with arthritis is calcium ascorbate, which is easily absorbed in the intestinal tract and less likely to cause diarrhea, which can occur if your dog takes too much vitamin C in one dose. Generally, puppies can take 250 to 500 mg daily, while 500 to 1,000 mg is safe for mature medium-size dogs and up to 2,000 mg is acceptable for giant breeds, according to Richard H. Pitcairn, DVM, author of *Dr. Pitcairn's Complete Guide to Natural Health for Dogs & Cats*.

Chapter 5

Atopic Dermatitis

Do you suffer with seasonal allergies? Are you allergic to indoor substances such as dust and pillow feathers? You are not alone, because about 10 to 15 percent of dogs also experience allergic reactions to pollens, house mites, and other allergens. But while people typically suffer with sneezing, itchy eyes, and a congested or runny nose, dogs respond mainly through their skin and react by scratching and licking, which is why doggie allergies often is a type of dermatitis involving skin inflammation and irritation. (See "Does My Dog Have Atopic Dermatitis?" on page 90.)

Dogs can suffer from several different kinds of dermatitis, but one of the most common types is atopic dermatitis. Also known as canine atopy, atopic dermatitis is a skin condition in which dogs have an inherited tendency (atopic) to develop specific antibodies when exposed to allergens that they inhale or that make contact with their skin. This form of dermatitis is second only to flea allergy dermatitis (see chapter 11, "Fleas and Ticks").

Signs of atopic dermatitis usually come on gradually, first affecting dogs in late summer or early fall in response to pollens typical of that time of year. Then dogs begin responding to pollens at other times of the year, and eventually they may also become sensitive to indoor allergens, such as house dust, mold, and feathers. As the years pass, the itching and scratching occur year round.

Part of the allergic reaction is the release of histamines, substances that the cells of the immune system release in response to allergens. The histamines then prompt inflammatory responses in the skin, nasal passages, and lungs that result in allergic symptoms.

DOES MY DOG HAVE ATOPIC DERMATITIS?

Dogs can begin to show signs of atopic dermatitis as early as three months of age, although typically they occur when dogs are one to three years old. For the majority of affected dogs, the symptoms include:

- itching
- scratching
- rubbing, especially the head or rolling on the ground
- licking, especially around the face, paws, and underarms
- sneezing and/or runny nose (known as allergic rhinitis).

Some dogs with atopic dermatitis develop an ear canal infection, which causes their ear flaps to become red and inflamed and a brown wax to accumulate in their ear canals. Infrequently, atopic dermatitis progresses to a more serious stage in which the dog develops deep scratches in the skin from itching and scratching and experiences scabs, hair loss, and bacterial skin infections. If you take care of atopic dermatitis early, you can prevent these symptoms.

Some breeds are more susceptible to atopic dermatitis than others, and include boxers, bulldogs, Dalmatians, English setters, golden retrievers, Irish setters, Labrador retrievers, Lhasa apsos, poodles, West Highland white terriers, and wire fox terriers, among others. However, any dog can be affected, including mixed breeds.

DIAGNOSING ATOPIC DERMATITIS

Diagnosing atopic dermatitis can be a challenge, because the symptoms mimic those of other allergic or skin conditions, especially flea allergy dermatitis, which affects the majority of dogs with canine atopy. Food allergies also are not uncommon among dogs and can accompany atopic dermatitis, contributing to the itching and scratching. Therefore, your veterinarian may suggest doing intradermal skin testing, which involves injecting minute amounts of various allergens into your dog and observing any skin reactions. This is done over a period of time and can be expensive.

Diagnosis of atopic dermatitis can be suspected based on your veterinarian's examination as well as your reported observations of your dog's history of allergic reactions. That's why it is important for you to keep notes on when signs of allergic reactions first occurred, the time of year they first appeared and when they reappeared, and how your dog reacted. Also note any changes you made in your dog's diet.

Atopic dermatitis rarely goes away by itself, nor does it often go into remission. Therefore, you need to find ways to manage it effectively. Short of removing your dog from all the allergens in his or her environment—which generally is not possible because dogs with atopic dermatitis are allergic to many different substances—there are various ways to treat this condition.

PLAYING "KEEP AWAY FROM ALLERGENS"

If your dog is allergic to the following allergens, here are some "keep away" hints:

(continued)

House Dust and House Dust Mites
- Keep your dog out of the rooms for several hours after you have vacuumed.
- Don't let your dog sleep on stuffed furniture (unless it his own, which then should be covered with either a plastic cover or a cloth cover that you wash often in hot water).
- Do not give your dog stuffed toys.
- Keep your dog in rooms that do not have carpeting.

Mold
- Keep your dog out of basements, crawl spaces under porches and decks, and greenhouses.
- Keep your dog indoors when you mow the lawn.
- Use a dehumidifier in the house and keep the filters clean and disinfected.

Pollens
- Keep your dog out of fields.
- Wipe your dog down with a damp towel or wash him after he has spent time in weeds or high grass.
- Keep your lawn cut short and weeds and brush cleared away.
- Allow your dog to stay indoors whenever possible during high pollen season

CONVENTIONAL TREATMENT

One conventional medical option for dogs with atopic dermatitis is a series of allergy shots, which can help dogs gradually build up resistance to the offensive allergens. This approach involves about nine to twelve months of shots, and dogs generally don't start to enjoy improvements in itching and scratching until after about six months of injections.

Other options include the use of medications such as corticosteroids and antihistamines to control or reduce itching. Corticosteroids (e.g., betamethasone, dexamethasone, hydrocortisone, methylprednisolone, prednisone, and prednisolone) are hormones that are effective at managing itching, but they also have serious side effects. If corticosteroids are used, they should be given at the lowest possible doses and only for a limited amount of time—no more than seven to ten days. Even when used for only a short time, corticosteroids can cause an increase in appetite and increased water intake and urination. Longer-term use can result in skin problems (seems counterproductive, doesn't it?), vision problems, damage to joints, diabetes, obesity, respiratory problems, hair loss, high blood pressure, and gastrointestinal issues. Antihistamines may help control itching and scratching in up to 40 percent of dogs with atopic dermatitis.

HOME REMEDIES

It's not uncommon for dogs to have several allergy and skin conditions occurring at the same time; that is, flea allergy along with atopic dermatitis, and/or food allergies. The symptoms for all three are similar, yet the causes are different, and so a combination of home remedies can best address both the causes and symptoms. These home remedies can be used along with conventional treatments; in fact, use of home remedies (especially diet) along with conventional approaches may significantly reduce or even eliminate your need for medications, if you have chosen to use them. Do consult your veterinarian before starting any type of treatment for your dog.

Diet

Changing your dog's diet is a key remedy for atopic dermatitis and associated skin conditions. A healthy diet can enhance the ability of the immune system to fight the allergens, reduce allergic responses, and help eliminate histamines. Therefore, if your dog is eating commercial kibble, make a switch to a diet that is as natural as possible (see chapters 2 "Is Dog Food Fit for Your Dog?" and 3 "What's for Dinner? Good Food for Your Dog"). A change in diet may make a significant difference in how your dog responds to allergens.

Keep in mind that dogs with atopic dermatitis may also have food allergies, and so they can benefit from a dietary change, especially a switch to homemade foods that are free of additives and preservatives and that also limit or avoid possible allergens. If you make a dietary change and try other remedies for atopic dermatitis and your dog is still not getting significant relief, then a food allergy may be playing a role. Even if your dog does not have food allergies, feeding her a natural diet is the healthiest choice for overall health.

Elimination Diet

Because atopic dermatitis and food allergies frequently occur together, an elimination diet can help dogs who continue to experience some symptoms even after they have switched to a natural diet and perhaps have taken medications as well. The list of the most common food allergens in dogs may surprise you, and here they are in the order of most offensive first: beef, dairy products, chicken, lamb, fish, chicken eggs, corn, wheat, and soy.

If you are thinking, *But these are the main ingredients found in dog food,* you are right, which is why identifying which food or foods your dog may be allergic to can be a challenge. However, once you discover the offending foods and remove them from your dog's diet, you will have significantly improved the quality of your dog's life. Here's how it's done.

- **Think of all the different foods your dog has ever consumed, both commercial dog food and people food.** Now choose one protein and one carbohydrate that your dog has never eaten before. These are the only two foods you will feed your dog for the next eight to twelve weeks. That's how long it will take before you see any significant improvement in symptoms. Some suggestions are turkey and sweet potato, fish and quinoa, or duck and brown rice.
- **During the elimination diet, do not give your dog any treats, table scraps, rawhide chews, or flavored medications.** Your dog also should not be allowed to roam, which may allow him access to garbage or other food sources.
- **An alternative to providing home-cooked dog food is to use specialized dog foods labeled "limited antigen" or "hydrolyzed protein."** Check the ingredients to see if your dog has had a negative reaction to any of the ingredients.
- **Once your dog's allergy symptoms have subsided significantly, you can add back one food item—for example, beef—for two weeks.** If your dog does not begin to experience allergy symptoms after the addition of beef, then you can add back another item for another two weeks. Anytime your dog shows symptoms, stop the latest food addition, wait until the symptoms subside, and then you can add yet another item.
- **Once you have identified which foods are safe for your dog and which ones are not, you can formulate a diet that includes the safe foods.**

- **Be sure the diet you choose is balanced with the right amount of vitamins, minerals, and other nutrients your dog needs.** This balance often can be achieved by adding vegetables and/or a nutritional supplement to your dog's meals. You can also consult with your veterinarian or a canine nutritionist to make sure your homemade dog foods contain all the necessary nutrients.

Omega-3 and Omega-6 Fatty Acids

Omega-3 fatty acids, which are found primarily in coldwater fatty fish in the form of EPA (eicosapentaenoic acid) and DHA (docosahexaenoic acid), can reduce inflammation and the impact of histamines that are released during an allergic reaction. EPA also fights inflammation by competing with the inflammation-promoting omega-6 fatty acid called arachidonic acid and reducing its harmful effects.

Not all omega-6 fatty acids promote inflammation, and your dog may benefit by taking one that actually helps reduce it. Gamma linolenic acid (GLA) has anti-inflammatory properties, and when it is taken as a supplement, much of it is converted to a substance called DGLA (dihomo-gamma-linolenic acid), which is the inflammation fighter. Like EPA, DGLA competes with arachidonic acid, and it also causes the release of a substance called prostaglandin E1, which inhibits the release of arachidonic acid from cells.

Therefore, you may want to include GLA with the omega-3s EPA and DHA to help treat atopic dermatitis. Most dogs respond to the benefits of omega-3 fatty acid supplements within about one month when they are taken daily. A suggested dose is 50 mg/kg/day of EPA and 35 mg/kg/day of DHA.

Omega-3s are very safe for dogs. When omega-3 fatty acids are used along with antihistamines or steroids, use of the drugs typically can be decreased or even stopped.

Limited research has been done on the effectiveness of omega-3 fatty acids on atopic dermatitis in dogs. A Colorado State University study included twenty-nine dogs who were given either flax oil, EPA plus DHA, or placebo daily for ten weeks. All the dogs that were given flax oil or EPA plus DHA improved, but not the dogs in the placebo group.

GLA is found in some plant-based oils, such as borage, black currant seed, and evening primrose oil. A typical dose is 8 mg per 10 to 25 pounds of body weight. Nutrients that help the body make the conversion from GLA to DGLA include vitamins C, B_3 (niacin), and B_6, along with magnesium and zinc. Look for GLA supplements that contain at least a few of these nutrients.

Biotin

Biotin is one of the B vitamins and is available as a supplement you can give your dog to help improve itchy, allergic skin. This nutrient is often used along with omega-3 fatty acids and GLA, and it has no side effects. Biotin is available as a powder that can be added to your dog's food. Use as directed on the label.

Bathing Hints

A dog with atopic dermatitis can be bathed about once every two weeks, although some dogs may need more frequent bathing, depending on the condition of their skin. Overbathing will remove the skin's natural oils and dry out the skin. When you give your dog a bath, use a mild, all-natural shampoo (hypoallergenic or colloidal oatmeal) or soap and use a 50-50 combination of white vinegar and water as the final rinse to restore the proper pH balance to the skin.

Other Remedies

- **Aloe vera.** The gel inside a succulent aloe vera leaf can be applied to irritated spots on your dog to provide some relief. Snip off the end or slice of leaf to release the gel and apply as needed.
- **Enzymes.** Since all organic allergens are proteins, and certain enzymes help with the breakdown (metabolism) of proteins into amino acids (which no longer have allergic powers), giving your dog an enzyme supplement may help with atopic dermatitis symptoms. In addition, the body starts a histamine response when the enzyme levels in the body are low, resulting in allergy symptoms. Therefore, the addition of enzymes (powdered plant enzymes are recommended) to your dog's food is suggested. Enzyme supplements for dogs are available and are dosed based on the amount of food you feed your dog. (See chapter 9, "Diarrhea," for more details on enzymes.)
- **Vitamin E.** This nutrient can be helpful both topically and internally. If your dog has some spots that are especially irritated from scratching, rub some vitamin E oil on those areas. For internal use, the suggested dose is 400 to 600 IU once or twice daily, depending on the size of your dog.

Chapter 6

Cognitive Dysfunction Syndrome (Doggie Dementia)

Grow old gracefully and with dignity: That's what many people say they want to do as they live through their golden years. But a harsh reality is that dementia strikes a great percentage of older people, and it can rob them of their ability to achieve that goal. The same mental robbery can happen to your dog. Doggie dementia—also known as cognitive dysfunction syndrome in dogs—is a real health challenge, and one that has been greatly underdiagnosed. But that is changing as more and more pet parents and veterinarians recognize the symptoms and are becoming aware of the advances being made in the identification and treatment of this age-related problem. Doggie dementia can be managed in a variety of ways, allowing you and your dog to have quality time together, even in his declining years.

WHAT IS DOGGIE DEMENTIA?

It's a mixed blessing that man's best friends naturally develop the same type of cognitive decline associated with Alzheimer's disease as people do. Dogs are considered by scientists to be natural models of Alzheimer's disease, and so the research on Alzheimer's disease may help both people and their dogs. In addition, a growing number of studies are being conducted specifically on the effects of dementia on dogs' behavior, motor skills, and social responsiveness, as well as on the impact of certain treatments.

As in people, doggie dementia is the gradual decline of cognitive functioning and is associated with the accumulation of substances in the brain called beta-amyloid peptide. These deposits, along with oxidative damage to brain cells, which progressively increases with age, can contribute to dementia. As in human medicine, improvements in nutrition and medical care have allowed our canine companions to live longer, and so they are more likely to experience the breakdown in brain functioning that accompanies aging.

DOES MY DOG HAVE DEMENTiA?

Here are some indications your dog may have dementia. If you notice one or more of these signs, keep track of them in a log, noting when they occur, how long they last, and how often they occur so you can discuss them with your veterinarian.

- **Disorientation.** This is one of the most common symptoms of doggie dementia, and it can show up in a number of ways. Dogs may go to a corner and stand there, headfirst, unable to decide what to do next. Some dogs stand on the wrong side (hinge side) of doors, waiting for them to open. When Buster, a thirteen-year-old Australian shepherd mix, started standing in corners, his pet parents were puzzled until friends told them the same thing had happened to their dog and a veterinarian had made a diagnosis of dementia. "At first I didn't know what to do when Buster stood in the corner," said Megan, Buster's pet mother, "and I felt really sad. So we started giving him more attention, even though sometimes he didn't seem to know us." Dogs with dementia may also stop responding to their name or commands that used to be familiar to them. However, if this is the only sign you observe, your dog may be experiencing hearing loss, so this possibility should be ruled out.

- **Changes in family interactions.** Dogs with dementia may walk away from family members and not greet them at the door like they used to. Some dogs tend to interact less with family members, while others suddenly don't want to leave their pet parent's side. If your Newfoundland mix Sadie suddenly seems to be hanging by your side a lot more than she used to and she's getting up in years, look for some of the other signs of doggie dementia as well.
- **Pacing.** Some dogs will pace or wander around the house or yard aimlessly. Dogs with dementia tend to engage more in such wandering behavior than in purposeful activity.
- **Loss of housetraining.** Dementia may cause dogs to forget their housetraining habits, and so you may find accidents in the house. You should remember that the dog is not urinating and defecating in the house on purpose. (Note: Medical problems such as gastrointestinal conditions or urinary tract infections should be ruled out.)
- **Loss of appetite.** Similar to elderly people, some senior dogs lose interest in food or forget to eat, even when the food is placed in front of them. Loss of appetite can be a sign of many other medical conditions as well (e.g., gastritis and dental problems), so look for other signs as well.
- **Barking.** A dog with dementia may bark frequently for no apparent reason. This can occur because she is confused or lost or does not recognize family members. It can be frustrating for pet parents, because telling the dog to stop can actually make her mental condition worse.
- **Sleep changes.** Dogs with dementia may sleep more than normal, sleep during the day and stay

awake at night, or display confusion at night when they used to sleep well.

DIAGNOSING DOGGIE DEMENTIA

Some of the symptoms associated with doggie dementia may be due to diseases or other medical conditions, such as side effects of drugs, organ failure, cancer, or the presence of an infection, so it is important for your dog to be examined by a veterinarian for these and other possible causes of your dog's dementia-like behaviors. It is also possible your dog could have dementia along with other physical problems that could be aggravating the mental decline.

No specific tests are available to identify cognitive dysfunction syndrome in dogs. Although a magnetic resonance imaging (MRI) scan may reveal some brain shrinkage, such an expensive test is rarely ordered unless a veterinarian suspects a brain tumor. A diagnosis of doggie dementia typically is given after a physical examination, identifying any other medical conditions that may be causing the symptoms (e.g., cancer, side effects of medications, and infections), and reviewing the dog's behaviors.

CONVENTIONAL TREATMENTS

A drug called selegiline, which is used in humans to treat Parkinson's disease, has been shown to relieve symptoms of cognitive dysfunction in some dogs. Selegiline works by prolonging the activity of a brain chemical (neurotransmitter) called dopamine, which is in short supply in dogs who have cognitive dysfunction. Selegiline (brand name Anipryl, specifically for dogs) is not effective for all dogs who have dementia, and it may also cause some side effects, although they tend to be mild. Those effects may include drowsiness, excessive drooling, diminished hearing, itching, shivering, vomiting, diarrhea, restlessness, repetitive movements, and licking. If your dog takes too much selegiline, her pupils may be slow to respond to changes in light and she may pant excessively. If these reactions occur, call your veterinarian immediately.

Older dogs are sometimes prescribed medications for other conditions, so before you give your dog selegiline, talk to your veterinarian. If your dog is taking meperidine, fluoxetine, tricyclic antidepressants, or ephedrine, these drugs can interact in a negative way with selegiline. Be sure to check with your veterinarian before using any of these drugs for your dog.

HOME REMEDIES

Although no pet parents want their dog to be affected by doggie dementia, the good news is some natural remedies have been shown to be helpful, and there is even scientific research to support their use. With that in mind, here are some home remedies you can try to help with cognitive dysfunction in your pooch.

Diet

Once again, a nutritious diet is all-important. If you haven't switched to a natural homemade food diet yet, it's not too late to start. However, if your dog is already demonstrating signs of dementia, changing her diet to one that includes new foods may be a challenge, since introducing new things to dogs who suffer with dementia can be confusing for the dog. (See "How to Help Your Dog with Dementia" on page 107.) Therefore, you will need to experiment with new foods gradually to see how they are received. You can, however, simultaneously use the other home remedies suggested in this section.

Since doggie dementia involves oxidative damage, it has been suggested that giving dogs antioxidants could be helpful, and a number of studies have supported this claim. For a group of beagles tested in a study published in May 2012, for example, eating a diet rich in antioxidants improved and maintained the dogs' cognition while also reducing oxidative damage. A full decade earlier, scientists at the University of California conducted studies in dogs and found that oxidative damage has a negative impact on cognitive function and that giving dogs antioxidants "can result in significant improvements." Including more foods high in antioxidants, such as vegetables and fruits as snacks, or including an antioxidant supplement in the food may be helpful.

Choline

Choline is a member of the B-complex vitamin family and is a water-soluble nutrient. Its main purpose in the body is to assist in the production of the neurotransmitter acetylcholine, which has a major role in brain functions such as memory, mood, and intelligence. Choline also is a key component of fat-containing structures in cell membranes, which themselves are made up almost entirely of fats. In particular, cell membranes contain fat-like molecules called phosphatidylcholine and sphingomyelin, both of which need choline. It so happens these molecules are abundant in the brain, so it's important to provide enough choline to keep these cells healthy. In fact, a low level or deficiency of acetylcholine is associated with dementia.

Dogs typically need only a minute amount of choline, and they get it readily from their diet. Foods rich in choline include beef, eggs, chicken, turkey, and some vegetables and legumes. However, as dogs get older, they are not able to process the choline from their food as well as they used to. When that happens, cognitive decline can develop.

Clinical studies have shown that when dogs take choline

supplements, pet parents can see some signs of improvement in cognitive functioning. If urinary incontinence is one of the signs of your dog's dementia (e.g., if Sadie has started peeing in the house), choline may help as it's has been shown to reduce this problem.

The suggested dose of choline for cognitive dysfunction is 50 to 100 mg daily for a dog that weighs 50 pounds. Choline is available as a single ingredient, but you can also find it in supplements that contain other B vitamins, all specially formulated for dogs.

Ginkgo biloba

Ginkgo biloba is an herb that is commonly referred to as an antiaging remedy and an herb that can help with memory in humans. However, there is some evidence it may help in dogs as well. Here's what one study showed.

In Germany, forty-two elderly dogs were given ginkgo extract at a daily dose of 40 mg per 10 kg (22 pounds) for eight weeks. At the end of just four weeks, a positive effect was already apparent. By the end of the study, the researchers reported that the "severity of the geriatric condition in dogs with a history of geriatric behavioural disturbances [which averaged 1 year] was significantly reduced." In fact, 36 percent of the dog were completely free of signs of dementia (disorientation, sleep/activity changes, behavior changes, general behavior, general physical condition/energy) by the end of the study.

Additional evidence comes from a study in aging beagles who were given a supplement specially formulated for cognitive problems in dogs (not available in the United States). Each capsule contained 50 mg ginkgo biloba extract, 25 mg phosphatidylserine, 20.5 mg vitamin B_6, and 33.5 mg natural vitamin E as d-alpha-tocopherol. One capsule was given for every 5 kilograms (about 11 pounds) of the dog's weight; therefore, a 25-pound dog was given two capsules daily for seventy days. The researchers used a memory test and found that memory and cognitive functioning improved in the dogs who took the supplement when compared with the dogs who did not.

Medium-Chain Triglycerides

Research has shown that long-term supplementation with medium-chain triglycerides (MCT) can improve cognitive function in aged dogs. This is an area of research that has shown some promise, and there are numerous studies to back up the claims that MCTs are beneficial for dogs who are experiencing cognitive decline.

Medium-chain triglycerides provide the brain with energy in the form of substances called ketones, which are substances the body produces when it burns fat for energy. In a study of beagles, one group of aged dogs was given a diet supplemented with 5.5 percent medium-chain triglycerides for eight months, and this group was compared with beagles who did not receive the supplement. All the dogs were evaluated for learning ability, attention, and similar tests.

The beagles who took the supplement had elevated levels of a ketone called beta-hydroxybutyrate, and these dogs performed significantly better on most of the cognitive tests than did the beagles who did not get the supplement. The authors of the study concluded that "brain function of aged dogs can be improved by MCT supplementation, which provides the brain with an alternative energy source."

Although medium-chain triglycerides appear to help with doggie dementia, currently there are no supplements specifically for dogs. However, MCT supplements for humans are readily available in liquid form, which makes it easy to give to your dog. Check with your veterinarian or canine nutritionist for the best dose for your dog.

HOW TO HELP YOUR DOG WITH DEMENTIA

I realize you cannot completely change your lifestyle, but if you are aware of a few things that can cause greater confusion for your dog with dementia, then you can take the appropriate steps to minimize her confusion and improve her quality of life and your life with your dog.

- ✓ **Keep the environment familiar.** Don't move furniture around and hold off on getting that new couch. Maintain the yard in the same way you have been; adding or removing lawn furniture, pools, and landscaping can be confusing for your dog, so keep it to a minimum.
- ✓ **Limit introducing new things to your dog.** This can include new toys, foods, people, and other animals.
- ✓ **Keep a routine.** This one step can be extremely important: Maintain the same times for feeding, walking, playtime in the yard, and sleeping.
- ✓ **Use simple, calm commands.** Long and/or loud commands can be frightening and confusing for your dog.
- ✓ **Keep playing.** Spend a short time each day interacting in a gentle, loving way with your dog.
- ✓ **Eliminate obstacles.** Dogs with dementia often have difficulty negotiating passageways that are cluttered and stairways. Steps may become a problem as well, so a ramp may be necessary.
- ✓ **Avoid using chemical flea and tick products.** Switch to natural remedies for these pests to avoid exposing your dog to the dangerous chemicals in these products.

Chapter 7

Dental Disease

A person's smile is often one of the first things people notice when meeting someone, especially if the smile is memorable—strikingly beautiful or a vision of poor dental health. Although dogs do "smile" in their own way, pet parents do not often have close-up moments with their dog's pearly whites unless they are taking a few moments on a regular basis to clean their dog's teeth. The lack of routine dental care is the main reason why periodontal disease is one of the most common problems veterinarians see in their practices.

The *State of Pet Health 2011 Report* noted the number one disorder among dogs is dental disease, affecting 78 percent of canines. The presence of dental disease is associated with more serious conditions, such as liver disease and kidney problems, and it can also have a significant impact on your dog's ability to chew and get proper nutrition. Therefore, maintaining good oral health for your dog is essential for his overall well-being.

DOES MY DOG HAVE DENTAL DISEASE?

The two dental problems most seen in dogs are gingivitis, a reversible condition that involves inflammation of the gums; and periodontitis, an inflammatory condition that affects the deeper structures of the teeth. If you keep a watchful eye on your dog's gums and teeth and have the teeth cleaned regularly, you will catch any early signs of dental disease and prevent it from progressing.

What signs indicate doggie dental disease? Here are signs of gingivitis and periodontitis.

- accumulation of tartar on the teeth along the gum line
- red, swollen gums that bleed when touched
- pawing the mouth
- not allowing anyone to touch his face or mouth
- swelling on the cheeks or below the eyes
- sneezing and/or runny nose
- bad breath (halitosis)
- painful chewing (The dog drops food while eating or turns her head to the side to chew on one side only.)
- excessive salivation
- loose teeth that eventually fall out
- weight loss (from an inability to eat).

Toy breeds and small dogs are more likely to develop dental disease than are larger dogs, because small dogs tend to have crowded teeth or teeth that are too big for their mouth. Dogs who groom themselves also have a greater risk of getting dental disease. However, any dog can develop problems with his teeth, especially if his diet is poor and/or his oral health is neglected.

GINGIVITIS

Gingivitis can develop in your dog's mouth when bacteria, especially streptococcus and actinomyces, accumulate between the teeth and gums, resulting in inflammation, irritation, and bleeding. To see if your dog has gingivitis, pull down gently on her jowls and look at the teeth and gum line.

Dogs with gingivitis have dental tartar (yellowish-brown plaque composed of food particles, bacteria, and calcium salts) along the gum line. The tartar can force the gums to pull away from the teeth, which in turn allows tiny pockets to form in the gums. When food particles and bacteria get into these pockets, inflammation and infections occur.

When plaque first forms, it is soft, so this is the best (and easiest) time to remove it. As the plaque turns hard, it is referred to as calculus. In dogs, most calculus accumulates on the upper premolars and molars. Some breeds, including poodles and smaller dogs, tend to develop gingivitis more readily than other breeds.

PERIODONTITIS

Periodontitis develops when gingivitis is left untreated. The tiny pockets in the gums become infected and inflamed and loosen the teeth, causing them to eventually fall out. A dog with periodontitis often finds it difficult to eat and may stare at his bowl, pick at his food, and shake his head while eating as he attempts to find a place in his mouth that does not hurt when he chews. Abscesses can form in the gums and rupture into the sinus cavities, spreading infection.

DIAGNOSING DENTAL DISEASE

Since the words "Open wide and say 'Ah'" don't work when examining a dog's mouth, your veterinarian will need to sedate your dog to do any more than a quick look into his mouth. If your veterinarian's poking and probing reveal gingivitis or periodontitis, she will likely do X-rays, since more than half of the symptoms of dental disease lie hidden under the gum line. Early stages of disease will show a loss of density and sharpness of the root of the teeth, while X-rays will reveal bone loss in more advanced disease.

CONVENTIONAL PREVENTION AND TREATMENT

Veterinarians recommend you have your dog's teeth cleaned, scaled, and polished at least once a year. In between, there are home remedies you can use to keep your dog's teeth and gums healthy and to help prevent and treat gingivitis should it develop. (See "Home Remedies" below.)

If your dog has gingivitis, your veterinarian may recommend professional cleanings with fluoride treatments two or three times a year. If the gingivitis progresses, your veterinarian may want to apply liquid antibiotics to your dog's gums to stimulate healing and prevent any further pockets from forming.

Dogs who develop periodontitis and who have infections may need to have one or more teeth removed. If the gums are severely diseased, portions may need to be removed as well. Antibiotics are typically prescribed for one to three weeks following any type of dental surgery. Once the dog is back at home, a solution of 0.2 percent chlorhexidine (an antiplaque antiseptic) can be applied to the teeth and gums every day with cotton balls or a syringe. Chlorhexidine can also be delivered to the mouth in a patch that is applied to the inside surface of the upper lip. The patch also contains nicotinamide (vitamin B_3), and this combination can help prevent tartar and control bad breath.

HOME REMEDIES

One of the main contributors to dental disease in dogs is inadequate nutrition, so one of the best home remedies for both prevention and treatment is a nutritious diet (see chapter 3). Among the other things you can do to avoid or manage dental disease is a home remedy you and your dog can participate in every day: brushing! Here are guidelines for brushing and caring for your dog's teeth and gums, as well as some other home remedies.

Brushing Your Dog's Teeth

The best way to support and maintain your dog's oral health is to brush her teeth every day. This may sound like a lot, but once you and your dog establish the habit, it can take little more time than it takes to brush your own teeth. In fact, a convenient way to develop the habit is to brush your dog's teeth immediately before or right after you do your own.

First, you need doggie toothpaste or gel. Although you may enjoy the light, minty taste of your toothpaste, the toothpastes made for humans contain ingredients that can cause stomach upset for your dog. Toothpastes and gels made for dogs typically contain chlorhexidine, hexametaphosphate, or zinc gluconate. If your dog has gingivitis, your veterinarian may recommend you use a toothpaste with fluoride—but do not use a human toothpaste with fluoride.

Next, you need a canine toothbrush or finger pads (finger cots). Admittedly, putting a toothbrush or your fingers into your dog's mouth may take some getting used to both for you and your dog, so it's important to use whatever tools are most comfortable and effective for both of you.

Toothbrushes designed for dogs are angled and shaped somewhat differently from brushes made for people, and they tend to be smaller and have very soft bristles. Some have different-size bristles on both ends of the brush. Finger cots are like glove fingers that have tiny bristles on them, essentially turning your finger into a toothbrush. Simply apply a small amount of toothpaste to the cot and gently brush your dog's teeth. Finger cot brushes tend to work best for larger dogs because they have larger mouths and it is easier to get your finger to all the teeth, especially in the back. A toothbrush tends to work better for smaller dogs because their mouths are smaller and it is more difficult to get your finger to the back of the mouth.

Naturally, you don't want your dog to bite you, nor do you want the tooth brushing experience to be an unpleasant one. So here are some tips:

- **Maintain a positive tone.** This is important from the first day you begin training for toothbrushing and every session thereafter. Praise your dog and do not overly restrain her. You want to establish tooth brushing as a positive event. While you are still training your dog to get used to tooth brushing sessions, have a reward ready for her after each session— either a favorite tasty treat or something she likes to do, such as play catch or run in the yard.
- **Keep each tooth brushing session short—no more than three to five minutes.**
- **Before you even attempt to use a toothbrush or finger cot, spend a few sessions letting your dog get used to the taste of the toothpaste by allowing her to lick it off your finger.** Many toothpastes made for dog have flavors like chicken or beef. Praise your dog after she licks the toothpaste. If she doesn't like the taste, you may need to try a different kind. (To avoid spending money on a brand your dog may not like, try sample sizes first.) Some toothpastes and gels contain baking soda or citrus flavors that some dogs do not tolerate well. It may take several days of just allowing your dog to lick the toothpaste before you are ready to try using a toothbrush or finger cot.
- **Once your dog accepts the toothpaste or gel, help her get familiar with having a toothbrush**

or finger cot placed in her mouth. Use a small amount of paste on the brush or finger cot and place it in your dog's mouth against the front teeth. Allow your dog to get used to this feeling—do not brush the teeth yet. Praise your dog.

- **After your dog has accepted the combination of toothpaste and brush (or finger cot), it's time to brush the teeth.** Lift the upper lip gently and place the toothbrush or finger cot at a 45-degree angle to the gum line and gently brush back and forth. You don't need to brush the back of the teeth (the side toward the tongue). Talk to your dog in a positive tone throughout the session. Don't forget the reward at the end.

- **If you only brush a few teeth each time, that's okay.** If you can get the left side one day, the middle the next day, and the right on the third day, just keep track and continue the cycle. At least you are getting the job done!

Coenzyme Q10

Coenzyme Q10 (CoQ10) is a potent antioxidant that can help reduce gum inflammation and redness, pain, and bleeding. There are two ways you can treat your dog with CoQ10: Give him an oral supplement or rub the liquid supplement on the gums. A typically recommended oral dose is 0.25 to 1.0 milligram per pound of body weight daily. Coenzyme Q10 supplements especially made for dogs are available, and if you use them, follow the package directions for dosing. If you use a liquid or capsule form of CoQ10 that you can mix with water, you can rub slightly diluted CoQ10 on your dog's gums. Coenzyme Q10 is very safe for dogs and does not cause side effects.

Extra Dietary Tips

In addition to a homemade diet, here are a few extra dietary tips that can help prevent tartar buildup and keep your dog's breath fresher.

- ✓ **Carrots.** After your dog has finished her meal, give her a raw carrot. Chewing on the carrot not only helps loosen particles that may have lodged between the teeth and gums, it also stimulates more saliva, which washes the food pieces away.
- ✓ **Coriander leaves.** Also known as cilantro, this herb contains citronellol, a natural antiseptic that can help reduce bad breath as well as heal and prevent mouth sores. Make a mild tea using coriander leaves, allow it to cool, and serve in your dog's water bowl. Not all dogs enjoy the taste, but it's worth a try. You can also try grinding coriander leaves and mixing them into the dog's toothpaste.
- ✓ **Parsley.** Prepare breath freshener by steeping several sprigs of parsley in boiled water. Allow the tea to cool, remove the parsley, and put the tea into your dog's water bowl. If your dog doesn't enjoy the parsley water, you can put the tea into a spray bottle and spritz it into her mouth.
- ✓ **Yogurt.** A little after-dinner treat that can work on the bacteria in your dog's mouth is plain (no sugars or fruits) low-fat yogurt with live cultures. A tablespoon or two is all she needs.

Other Home Remedies

The following herbal remedies can be helpful if your dog has had dental work and his gums are irritated or inflamed. Use a cotton swab or soft cloth to apply these herbal remedies.

✓ **Calendula.** Also known as pot marigold, calendula is a common plant whose flower is used as an herbal remedy. Rub a tincture of calendula directly on your dog's gums to facilitate healing, reduce inflammation, and stop bleeding.

✓ **Echinacea.** If your dog has infected teeth, swabbing her gums with tincture of echinacea can help fight the infection and in turn reduce inflammation. Echinacea is one of the most popular herbs used to fight infections and has a history of use in both humans and animals.

✓ **Oregon grape.** The antibacterial properties of Oregon grape can help fight infection. Application of tincture of Oregon grape to your dog's gums may also help promote new gum tissue growth.

Chapter 8
Diabetes

The prevalence of diabetes is rising—and not just in people. Diabetes in dogs is a growing concern, but the good news is that, similar to diabetes in people, the disease can be managed at home.

According to the *State of Pet Health 2011 Report*, which includes medical information from 2.1 million dogs and nearly 450,000 cats, an analysis of pet health trends over five years found a 46 percent rise in canine diabetes since 2005. It's estimated that diabetes affects one in every 160 dogs in the United States. About 70 percent of dogs with diabetes are older than seven years when they are diagnosed, and the disease is about three times more common in females than in males.

Certain breeds are at higher risk for diabetes, including Australian terriers, bichons frises, cairn terriers, fox terriers, German shepherds, golden retrievers, keeshonds, miniature pinschers, miniature schnauzers, poodles, pulis, Samoyeds, schnauzers, Siberian huskies, and spitzes. However, diabetes can affect any dog or any breed.

TYPES OF DIABETES IN DOGS

The two types of diabetes in dogs are diabetes insipidus and diabetes mellitus. Diabetes insipidus is characterized by a lack of an antidiuretic hormone called vasopressin, whose job is to control the kidneys' absorption of water. This type is much less common than diabetes mellitus, which is characterized by insulin deficiency and is also the more dangerous type of diabetes in dogs. Of the two types of diabetes mellitus, type 1 and type 2, the former is much more common in dogs. This chapter focuses on type 1 diabetes.

Type 1 diabetes develops when there is insufficient production of insulin by the islet cells in the dog's pancreas. Some dogs may have a genetic predisposition for this lack of insulin. A deficiency of insulin results in high blood sugar (hyperglycemia) and high levels of sugar in the urine (glycosuria). Lots of sugar in the urine causes diabetic dogs to pee large amounts, which in turn leads to dehydration and the urge to drink large volumes of water.

DOES MY DOG HAVE DIABETES?

The classic symptoms of diabetes in dogs mimic those in people: increased urination, weight loss despite normal or even increased food intake, and excessive thirst. You may also notice that your dog's breath has a "sweet" odor. In more advanced cases of diabetes, dogs experience vomiting, dehydration, hair loss, weakness, lethargy, loss of appetite, and coma.

Most dogs with diabetes develop cataracts within six months of diagnosis, and about 80 percent have the eye condition within sixteen months. The risk of getting cataracts tends to increase as dogs get older, regardless of how well their sugar levels are controlled. Cataracts are the leading cause of blindness in dogs.

Your veterinarian can perform a few simple tests for sugar (glucose) levels in the blood and urine to determine if your dog has diabetes. Other test results that can identify diabetes are elevated liver enzymes and/or cholesterol and/or triglycerides, an enlarged liver, protein and/or ketones (by-products of fatty acids after they are metabolized in the liver and kidneys) in the urine, and low phosphorus in the blood.

Over time, dogs with diabetes can develop complications, such as kidney problems (diabetic nephropathy), urinary tract infections, infections of the mouth and gums (see chapter 7, "Dental Problems"), liver disease, pancreatitis (inflamed pancreas), and hyperlipidemia (high triglyceride levels). These complications can be improved as blood sugar levels are managed.

WHY DO DOGS GET DIABETES?

A common misconception is that dogs get diabetes if they get fat. Although being overweight or obese is a major factor in doggie diabetes, it is not the cause. Being overweight can contribute to insulin resistance, which then makes it more difficult to manage diabetes in dogs. Dogs who are obese are also at risk for pancreatitis, which can lead to diabetes.

An estimated 50 percent of dogs with diabetes are believed to develop the disease because of damage to their pancreases due to autoimmune disorders that could themselves be caused by genetics and environmental factors. One theory is that many cases of doggie diabetes are associated with overstimulation of the immune system from environmental assaults, such as vaccinations and processed foods (again, the importance of natural, unprocessed food needs to be emphasized).

About 30 percent of diabetes in dogs may be the result of an inflamed pancreas (chronic pancreatitis), while the remaining 20 percent can develop insulin resistance from Cushing's disease (hyperadrenocorticism, in which the body produces excessive amounts of glucocorticoid hormone, which is involved in carbohydrate metabolism), elevated growth hormone levels, or prolonged use of steroids.

Regardless of the cause, doggie diabetes can be managed, but it does take extra effort on the part of pet parents.

DIAGNOSING DIABETES IN DOGS

You can help your veterinarian with the diagnosis if you take notes about any symptoms you notice, when they started, and how long they have been going on. Along with asking about these symptoms, your veterinarian will also examine your dog to rule out other possible health conditions as well as test your dog's urine for glucose and ketones and her blood for glucose concentration. Diabetes is diagnosed only when glucose is detected in both the urine and the blood at a constantly high concentration.

CONVENTIONAL TREATMENT

Dogs with diabetes can have a lifespan similar to that of dogs without the disease if they receive proper treatment. The riskiest time is during the first six months after diagnosis and as treatment begins, because it takes some time to regulate blood sugar levels properly. This can be a stressful time for both you and your dog, so try to be patient.

Dogs with diabetes require insulin, and that means daily injections. So far, no oral drugs for diabetes have been developed for dogs. However, it's important to note that home remedies, including diet and supplements, can make managing blood sugar levels easier.

It typically takes some experimentation to find the type of insulin that best fits a dog's needs because the degree of failure of the pancreas differs for each dog. Insulin comes in short-, intermediate-, and long-acting forms, and often it is necessary to use a mixture of insulins to get the best results. Both recombinant human insulin and porcine (derived from pigs) insulin are most like the insulin dogs produce naturally, so these are the forms recommended.

Insulin is usually given two times a day, and it is best to

give it immediately after the dog eats. If a dog is given insulin before he or she eats and then refuses to eat, the insulin's effects could be dangerous. Your veterinarian will explain how to give insulin injections to your dog and how to monitor urine glucose levels using paper test strips.

HOME REMEDIES

Diet, Diet, Diet

If your canine companion has diabetes, not only is the composition of the food he or she eats important, but the timing of the meals is critical as well. You might call it the "same" approach: Feed your dog the same amount of the same type of food (this doesn't mean the exact same food, however, just the same type), and provide the food at the same time each day, preferably eight or twelve hours apart. Some dogs need a snack in between to prevent sugar levels from falling too low, a condition called hypoglycemia.

The "same" approach is critical because it helps your dog maintain a steady blood sugar level and works along with the insulin injections. Beyond that, however, you and your veterinarian will need to work together to identify the best diet for your dog, as there is no standard diet for dogs with diabetes, and few nutritional studies have been done on dogs who have diabetes. Each dog's dietary needs vary greatly, depending on factors such as body weight, amount of exercise the dog gets, the presence of any other medical conditions, and what foods the dog likes.

That said, here are some points to consider when deciding how to feed your diabetic dog. Talk these points over with your vet:

- **How much carbohydrates should my dog eat?**
  The amount of carbohydrates in your dog's diet is

important because any change in carbohydrates can have an impact on the amount of insulin your dog will need. Identifying the amount of carbs will likely be a matter of trial and error, so be patient. Foods that are low on the glycemic scale (e.g., most fruits and vegetables, some whole grains, and legumes) are best because they release glucose slowly and steadily into the bloodstream. Medium-glycemic foods, such as whole wheat, potatoes, and brown rice, should only be used in moderation, while high-glycemic foods (e.g., white rice, white bread, pasta, and sugars) should be avoided. A dog that does not do well on a low-carb diet will need more carbohydrates, which means the percentage of protein and/or fat will need to be reduced.

- **Does my diabetic dog need lots of fiber?** Fiber, which is the part of plant foods the body cannot digest, helps slow the digestion of carbohydrates and the release of glucose, so it plays a significant role in diabetes. Dogs with diabetes who eat a diet that is high in fiber experience less fluctuations in blood sugar levels. Most carbohydrates contain some fiber, and some are better sources of fiber than others. Commercial dog foods typically contain fiber.
- **How much fat should be in my dog's diet?** Most dogs with diabetes do well on a diet that is low in fat. And because many dogs with diabetes are also overweight, it's important to avoid weight gain.
- **How much protein does my dog need?** Typically, protein should make up 40 to 60 percent of your dog's diet.
- **Does the diet provide adequate nutrition?** Regardless of which balance of carbs, protein, and fat you find works best for your diabetic dog, the bottom line is the diet should meet your dog's nutritional needs (see chapter 1).

- **Can my dog have treats?** Most dogs enjoy treats, and dogs with diabetes are no exception. In fact, you may need treats to help balance blood sugar levels or as a reward after an insulin shot. Just make sure the treats are nutritious and appropriate; that is, choose crunchy vegetables such as carrot sticks, raw string beans, or snap peas. Avoid treats that are high in carbohydrates or sugar (e.g., soft or moist foods and treats), those that contain propylene glycol or similar chemicals, and dehydrated meats that are made in China. You can make your own dried meat or poultry treats by cutting the meat into ultrathin slices and placing them in a food dehydrator or baking them in a slow oven (275 to 300°F) until they get crunchy.
- **Are there special foods that can help my dog with diabetes?** Try including these vegetables in your dog's diet as part of the carbohydrate requirement: green beans (the pods contain substances related to insulin), dandelion greens, Jerusalem artichoke, and winter squash. (See also "Garlic: Safe or Toxic?" on page 62.)

Here are two homemade recipes that may be suitable for dogs with diabetes. Consult your veterinarian or canine nutritionist to see if they meet the needs of your dog.

Diabetes Recipe #1

$\frac{1}{2}$ cup lean beef or chicken, cooked
$2\frac{3}{4}$ cups cooked brown rice, barley, or oats
$\frac{1}{4}$ cup chopped broccoli, carrots, green beans, or sweet potatoes
1 medium egg, lightly scrambled
Daily multivitamin/mineral supplement and calcium as recommended by your veterinarian

If using the beef, pour off any fat from cooking. Combine all ingredients.

Diabetes Recipe #2

$1/4$ lb ground lean beef
$1/2$ cup farmer cheese
2 cups cooked sliced or chopped carrots
2 cups mixed frozen vegetables (cooked)
$1 1/2$ teaspoon dicalcium phosphate (check with your veterinarian to see if your dog needs this supplement)

Cook the beef until lightly brown and then pour off the fat. Add the remaining ingredients, including any nutritional supplements. Makes about $1 3/4$ pounds. Feed $2/3$ pound to a 10-pound dog, 1 pound to a 20-pound dog, and $1 3/4$ pound to a 40-pound dog.

Weight Control and Exercise

Weight control is intimately related to diet and exercise, but it's worth a separate section because achieving and maintaining a healthy weight is so critical in dogs who have diabetes, and overweight/obesity is a significant problem among diabetic dogs. Dogs who are too heavy are usually resistant to the effects of insulin. If you can help your dog drop excess pounds and bring him or her to a normal, healthy weight, you will likely also be able to reduce the amount of insulin your dog needs, improve stamina and exercise capacity, and improve your dog's quality of life.

Although physical exercise can reduce insulin resistance and the need for insulin, too much activity can cause blood sugar levels to drop too low, causing hypoglycemia. You can apply the "same" approach to exercise as you do to food: same amount of exercise each day, done at the same time.

Generally, it is best to provide exercise for your dog (walking, playing catch) for 20 to 30 minutes before the evening meal, followed by the insulin injection. If you and your dog decide to go for an unexpected long hike or other type of extra exercise, remember that extra activity will reduce your dog's need for insulin. You may be able to use half the amount or skip a dose after vigorous exercise to avoid hypoglycemia brought on by exercise.

Brewer's Yeast

Brewer's yeast is an excellent source of chromium, an essential trace mineral that helps the body maintain normal blood sugar levels, improve glucose tolerance, and thus reduce the amount of insulin your dog may need. Do not confuse brewer's yeast with nutritional yeast, baker's yeast, or torula yeast, all of which are low in chromium. Brewer's yeast is made from a fungus called *Saccharomyces cerevisiae* and is also a good source of protein, selenium, and the B-complex vitamins, which help break down carbohydrates, fats, and protein and provide the body with energy. A suggested dose of brewer's yeast is one teaspoon to one tablespoon, depending on the size of your dog, with each meal.

WHAT YOU SHOULD KNOW

Although early research suggested the use of glucosamine in dogs with diabetes might raise blood sugar levels, subsequent studies have come to different conclusions. If you give your diabetic dog glucosamine for arthritis or other inflammatory conditions, it's a good idea to monitor blood sugar levels after starting the supplement—just to make sure!

Other Home Remedies

- **Fenugreek.** Numerous studies in dogs have shown that fenugreek seeds or components added to the diet of dogs with diabetes lowers cholesterol and reduces high blood glucose. Fenugreek is available in supplements specifically for dogs. A typical dose for diabetes is 5 to 30 grams with each meal or 15 to 90 grams per day, depending on the size of your dog. If you use a tincture, 3 to 4 ml taken up to three times a day is suggested.
- **Garlic.** In human studies, garlic has been shown to reduce blood sugar levels and animal studies have revealed that it can increase insulin, but whether these benefits apply to dogs is not known. However, the addition of a small amount of garlic (½ clove to 2 cloves minced per day, depending on the size of your dog) could be beneficial.
- **Vitamin E.** Use of vitamin E may reduce your dog's need for insulin, control blood sugar levels, and improve insulin activity. A suggested dose is 25 IU to 200 IU per day, depending on the dog's size.

Chapter 9

Diarrhea

Although diarrhea is not a pleasant topic, the passage of loose, watery, unformed stools is a common symptom among dogs and one that most pet parents encounter at one time or another. Fortunately, most cases of doggie diarrhea are not serious and can be handled easily at home with some tender loving care and homemade remedies, which we discuss later in this chapter.

Sometimes, however, diarrhea is more serious, depending on the cause, certain characteristics of the diarrhea, and how long it lasts. Diarrhea can even be life threatening, so it's important to identify if your dog is experiencing dangerous diarrhea so she can be treated appropriately and promptly. Therefore, let's take a closer look (so to speak) at doggie diarrhea.

SERIOUS DIARRHEA

Here are the danger signs that should send you and your dog to the veterinarian as soon as possible:

- **You suspect your dog has eaten something toxic.** If possible, write down the name of the product or bring the label or item with you to the veterinarian's office so the doctor will know what poison your dog has ingested
- **Your dog has a fever.**

- **Your dog's gums are pale or yellow.**
- **Your dog looks bloated.**
- **The diarrhea is black, looks tarry, or is bloody.**
- **Your dog seems to be in pain.**
- **Your dog is vomiting.**
- **The diarrhea continues for more than twenty-four hours.**
- **Your dog is dehydrated** (see below).

Because any degree of diarrhea can be especially dangerous if it affects young puppies or elderly dogs, it is best to treat such cases of diarrhea as a serious health matter.

IS MY DOG DEHYDRATED?

Here are some signs that your dog is dehydrated:

- **Gums.** Healthy gums should be wet, reflective, and slippery; a dehydrated dog has sticky, dull gums.
- **Capillary refill time.** This is a fancy term for something that is easy to check. Gently press a finger against your dog's gums until the spot becomes white. Release and watch how long it takes for the gums to return to a pinkish color. If it does not happen immediately, your dog is likely dehydrated.
- **Skin.** Check your dog's skin elasticity: Grasp the loose skin over your dog's shoulders and lift it up as far as it will stretch and then release it. If the skin does not return immediately into place, then your dog is probably dehydrated.

- **Eyes.** Dogs who are dehydrated may have sunken eyes.

TYPES AND CAUSES OF DIARRHEA

Diarrhea in dogs can occur in one of two forms: acute or chronic. Acute diarrhea is by far the more common type, so we'll discuss it first.

Acute Diarrhea

Acute diarrhea is so named because it comes on suddenly and typically resolves within twenty-four to seventy-two hours, but may last as long as a week. If your dog has acute diarrhea, he may vomit once or twice along with the loose stools. Both the diarrhea and vomiting are nature's way of eliminating something that is irritating the dog's gastrointestinal system. Basically, dogs with acute diarrhea act somewhat like you would if you had a short bout of diarrhea: a little off your game, but still able to function pretty well.

Acute diarrhea can be triggered by a number of factors. For example:

- **Dietary mistakes.** Although eating garbage, dirt, grass, paper, or your favorite shoes are dietary mistakes to you, your dog probably enjoyed herself, since she wasn't aware diarrhea might be the result. Dietary mistakes are among the most common reasons for doggie diarrhea.
- **Intestinal parasites.** The presence of worms in the intestinal tract is another common cause of diarrhea, especially in puppies. Worms can cause

either acute or chronic diarrhea and are discussed in detail in chapter 17.

- **Stress.** Changes in a dog's life can be emotionally and/or physically stressful, and the stress may show up as diarrhea. If you have moved recently, added a new member to the household (e.g., a baby, another dog, a cat), left the dog in a kennel while you went on vacation, or switched from day shift to night shift, these are just a few examples of situations that are stressful for some dogs. The death of another dog in the home also may cause stress.
- **Intentional dietary changes.** If you switch from one dog food brand to another or if you start your dog on a homemade diet plan (hurray!), he may experience some diarrhea. However, loose stools can be avoided or greatly minimized if you make any dietary changes gradually by incrementally adding the new food while phasing out the former food.
- **Medications.** Use of certain medications, especially antibiotics, dewormers, and nonsteroidal anti-inflammatory drugs, may cause diarrhea.

Chronic Diarrhea

Chronic diarrhea is the presence of loose, watery, and/or unformed stools that occurs for a prolonged time (weeks) either every day or nearly every day. There may be some normal days in between days of diarrhea. Dogs with chronic diarrhea frequently have mucus-coated or bloody stools.

Chronic diarrhea is dangerous because your dog can lose a significant amount of nutrients and fluids, which can result in dehydration, malnutrition, and weight loss, and place the immune system under a great deal of stress. Because the intestinal tract is compromised, your dog can become toxic, since about 25 percent of the body's detoxification mechanisms are in the intestines.

Causes of chronic diarrhea can include:

- **Intestinal parasites.** Whipworms are the most common culprit (see chapter 17).
- **Bacterial or protozoan infections.** Among the more common of these infections are giardiasis (an infection of the small intestine by the protozoa giardia) and the bacteria clostridium, which are a common cause of diarrhea.
- **Food intolerance.** In cases of food intolerance, dogs who cannot tolerate certain foods, including beef, chicken, corn, fish, gravies, pork, soy, spices, and some commercial dog foods, can react to these foods by developing diarrhea. (Food intolerance differs from food allergy, which is associated with dermatitis and can cause vomiting.) Some adult dogs are lactose intolerant and cannot digest milk and milk products, which can also lead to diarrhea. Unless the diet is changed, the diarrhea can be chronic.
- **Intestinal disorders.** These include inflammatory bowel disease, colitis, and irritable bowel syndrome. A veterinarian will need to conduct tests to determine if any of these disorders are causing the diarrhea. One clue is stool with red blood or mucus, which suggests colitis, a condition characterized by an acute or chronic inflammation of the membrane that lines the colon.
- **Leaky gut syndrome.** Also known as intestinal permeability, this condition is characterized by damage to the small intestine in which there are spaces between the cells in the intestinal lining that allow pieces of partially digested food, toxins, and bacteria to escape from the intestines into the bloodstream. Chronic diarrhea is only one sign of leaky gut syndrome, which can be caused by a variety of factors, including a high-carbohydrate diet,

use of antibiotics or nonsteroidal anti-inflammatory drugs, and parasites, among other causes.
- **Organic diseases.** These may include liver disease, thyroid disease, and kidney disease. Although they are not nearly as common as dietary causes of diarrhea, they still should be considered.

DIAGNOSING DIARRHEA

You can help your veterinarian in the diagnosis of your dog's diarrhea if you provide the following information:

- ✓ **when the diarrhea started.** Acute diarrhea comes on suddenly and typically resolves within a day or two, while chronic diarrhea usually comes on gradually and can persist for weeks, or it can have an on-off pattern over a prolonged period of time.
- ✓ **any possible precipitating events or circumstances** (e.g., the dog is on medication or taking supplements, the dog's diet has been changed recently)
- ✓ **number of bowel movements your dog has had**
- ✓ **description of the diarrhea** (color, consistency, odor).
- ✓ **how your dog is acting** (e.g., listless, in pain, not eating).

This information will help your veterinarian determine if the diarrhea originated in the small bowel or the large bowel, which in turn will help her determine how to treat your dog. Your veterinarian will also collect information on your dog's medical history (including vaccinations and the use of dewormers and other medications), conduct a physical examination, and recommend a fecal flotation test, which checks for parasites such as worms.

If your dog is displaying signs of illness, your veterinarian may order a complete blood count, chemistry panel, and/or other blood tests. X-rays can be ordered if your veterinarian suspects a tumor or structural problem, while imaging tests such as ultrasound may also be helpful.

CONVENTIONAL TREATMENT

For most cases of acute diarrhea, home remedies are sufficient and even recommended. For more serious cases of diarrhea, the treatment depends on the cause. For example, diarrhea associated with a worm infestation will require therapies to eliminate the worms (see chapter 17, "Worms [Intestinal Parasites]"). Antibiotics may be prescribed if a bacterial infection is the cause of diarrhea, while a diagnosis of leaky gut syndrome will require a change in diet (to eliminate allergic reactions to foods) and restoration of a favorable bacteria balance in the intestinal tract using probiotics.

Perhaps the most common medication given to dogs who have diarrhea is one you are probably familiar with: Pepto-Bismol, which is bismuth subsalicylate and in the class of medications called antidiarrheals. Bismuth subsalicylate works by decreasing the flow of fluids and electrolytes into the bowel, reducing inflammation in the intestinal tract, and possibly killing any microorganisms that can cause diarrhea.

Although bismuth subsalicylate is safe for dogs, you should still check with your veterinarian before giving your dog this drug. Pepto-Bismol is one of the few drugs that is recommended for both people and dogs. It soothes the stomach and intestinal lining and can help relieve diarrhea that has been caused by something your dog ate. The typical dose is 0.5 to 1 ml of Pepto-Bismol per pound of body weight, and it should be given every six to eight hours.

To avoid getting the "pink bath"—which can happen when you give your dog liquid Pepto Bismol and she immediately shakes her head and sends the pink stuff flying—use a plastic syringe to squirt the medication into the back of her mouth. Pepto-Bismol is also available in tablet form.

Pepto-Bismol can cause side effects, the most common of which is black-colored stools. Some dogs do not tolerate silicates, in which case Pepto-Bismol will not be effective. Another medication for vomiting and diarrhea, called loperamide (Immodium), is safe for dogs. A typical dose is one teaspoon every four to six hours for every 20 pounds of body weight.

HOME REMEDIES

Your dog can likely be treated at home if he has mild acute diarrhea and does not meet any of the criteria for serious diarrhea listed at the beginning of this chapter. Still, it is best to consult with your veterinarian before starting any treatment options.

Diet

If your dog has acute diarrhea, the most important step you can take is to withhold all food for twenty-four to forty-eight hours so your dog's gastrointestinal tract can take a break. To prevent dehydration, make sure plenty of freshwater is available. Here are some other dietary recommendations:

✓ **Along with plain water, also give your dog a meatless broth.** You can make this using a variety of vegetables (no onions) and rice, but only give your dog the liquid. (Hint: If you don't use the vegetables and rice for yourself, you can freeze them for later use for a homemade dog food recipe, when your dog is feeling better.)

✓ **Once the diarrhea has stopped, begin a bland diet consisting of ground turkey with plain canned pumpkin or plain mashed sweet potato.** Feed this mixture (50:50) in small amounts three to five times a day. Pumpkin and sweet potato are easily digested and are good sources of fiber.

✓ **Put your dog on a "standard" bland diet.** Some veterinarians suggest a diet consisting of boiled hamburger and rice. However, hamburger is typically too fatty and the rice may cause digestive problems, so this approach is not recommended.

✓ **Keep your dog on the bland diet for several days after the diarrhea has resolved and then gradually return to his normal diet.** This is also a great time to gradually transition to a homemade dog food diet.

Enzymes

The pancreas naturally produces enzymes that are used for digesting carbohydrates (amylase), fats (lipase), and proteins (proteases). Additional enzymes can be provided by your dog's food, although commercially processed foods typically change the nutrients in the food and destroy enzymes.

When a dog has diarrhea, especially chronic diarrhea, the intestinal tract is under a great deal of stress. If you provide your dog with extra enzymes in the form of a supplement, they can support the intestinal cells and help them recover while also assisting in your dog's digestion and the absorption of nutrients from her food.

Enzymes are beneficial for dogs who have diarrhea associated with food allergies, bowel disease (especially inflammatory bowel disease), leaky gut syndrome, infections, use of medications (antibiotics in particular), stress, and poor diet. In fact, enzymes are recommended for any dog who is eating a commercial dog food.

When choosing enzyme supplements for your dog, look for plant enzymes rather than pancreatic enzymes, because those derived from plants are more active and also contain the enzyme cellulase, which is an additional aid to digestion. Pancreatic enzymes are derived from cadaver cows and pigs, are not viable in the stomach, and are incapable of breaking down fiber and certain carbohydrates.

Enzymes for dogs are available in pill and powder form, and the latter is much easier to use. Just sprinkle it on your dog's food: The food must be at room temperature and not warm or hot, because enzymes are rendered inactive by heat. Follow the recommended dose on the product, which is typically determined by the amount of food you give to your dog.

Dog enzyme products usually contain various enzymes, because different enzymes digest certain types of carbohydrates, proteins, and fats. Therefore, you want a supplement that contains a variety of enzymes, which may include proteases (there are several kinds), amylase, peptidase, alpha-galactosidase, beta-galactosidase, diastase, lipase, cellulase, pectinase, phytase, hemicellulase, and bromelain.

Probiotics

Not all bacteria are bad, and probiotics are an example of beneficial or good bacteria. The use of live beneficial bacteria has been shown to be effective in managing diarrhea in both dogs and humans. When you give your dog probiotics, the bacteria colonize in the intestinal tract, helping to maintain a harmonious balance between "good" and "bad," disease-causing bacteria. Probiotics accomplish this by producing short-chain fatty acids, which interfere with the growth and activity of harmful bacteria, like those that cause diarrhea, irritable bowel syndrome, and intestinal inflammation. Because diarrhea can kill good bacteria, providing more beneficial bacteria in the form of probiotics can counteract this destruction.

Probiotics can be especially helpful for dogs who have taken antibiotics, because these drugs kill bad and good bacteria at the same time. Giving your dog probiotics after a treatment course of antibiotics can assist in restoring the bacterial balance in her intestinal tract and help prevent or eliminate diarrhea.

There are many different species and strains of beneficial bacteria that belong to five main categories (genera): *Bacillus, Bifidobacterium, Enterococcus, Lactobacillus*, and *Streptococcus*. Among the specific strains that have been found to be helpful in dogs with diarrhea are *Enterococcus faecium* (strain SF68), *Bacillus coagulans, Bifidobacterium animalis* (strain AHC7), and *Lactobacillus acidophilus*.

You can find probiotic supplements specially for dogs in pills, powder, and liquid form. Probiotic products typically contain more than one species and/or strain of beneficial bacteria. Be sure to follow label instructions concerning storage of probiotics, because some brands contain species that require refrigeration to remain viable. Probiotics that are freeze-dried may last longer than products that are powdered or must be refrigerated. Also check the expiration date on any probiotic supplements.

Little is known about effective dosages of probiotics for dogs with diarrhea, but because beneficial bacteria are safe, you don't have to worry about giving your dog too much. In fact, probiotics are measured by colony forming units (CFUs), and typical doses are in the hundreds of millions. Follow dosing recommendations on the bottle. If you use a probiotic product for humans, give the full recommended dose to your dog if she weighs 40 pounds or more, and reduce the dose if she weighs less.

PROBIOTIC STUDIES FOR DOGS WITH DIARRHEA

Several studies have examined the benefits of probiotics for dogs with diarrhea. One involved thirty-six dogs who had acute diarrhea or acute diarrhea and vomiting. All were given either probiotics (*Lactobacillus acidophilus*, *Pediococcus acidilactici*, *Bacillus subtilis*, *Bacillus licheniformis*, or *Lactobacillus farciminis*) or placebo. The dogs who took the probiotics experienced diarrhea for a significantly shorter time (1.3 days) compared with dogs given placebo (2.2 days).

In an earlier study conducted in Ohio, investigators looked at the effect of *Bifidobacterium animalis* strain AHC7 in dogs who had acute diarrhea. Eighteen dogs were given placebo and thirteen received the probiotic. The dogs given the probiotic got relief from diarrhea in an average of 3.9 days compared with 6.6 days for dogs who received placebo.

Slippery Elm

Even the name "slippery elm" sounds soothing, doesn't it? This herb can help protect the mucous membranes and ease the irritation in the intestinal tract. To prepare a slippery elm remedy, mix one teaspoon of slippery elm powder with one cup of water, bring it to a boil, and let it simmer for 2 to 3 minutes. After the tea has cooled, give your dog the remedy four times a day based on size: 1 teaspoon per dose for small dogs, 1 to 2 tablespoons per dose for medium dogs, and 3 to 4 tablespoons per dose for large dogs.

Chapter 10

Ear Problems

Do your dog's ears smell? Does your dog rub his ears on the carpet or on the furniture? Has your dog been scratching his ears lately? These are all signs of ear problems, many of which can be very minor and easily resolved, while others can be more serious but still treatable. Once you and your veterinarian decide the type of ear problem you dog has, you can choose appropriate home remedies.

Ear infections are among the most common health issues that affect dogs. One reason dogs are susceptible to ear infections has to do with anatomy: A dog's ear canals are positioned downward and then go horizontal, away from the ear opening. Therefore, if anything gets into the ear—even water—it can get stuck in the ear canal and promote infection.

Floppy ears is another anatomical reason dogs get ear infections. Dogs who have ears that are erect or that do not fold over completely are less likely to get ear infections because floppy ears keep the inside of the ear flap and the ear canal warm and moist, which is a perfect breeding ground for bacteria and yeast/fungi.

DOES MY DOG HAVE EAR PROBLEMS?

Indications that your dog has ear problems include the following:

- **Smelly ears.** This may be accompanied by the presence of waxy buildup or a discharge (see below).
- **Discharge from the ears.** This is usually in the form of black particles or is yellow and pasty.
- **Dog shakes his head from side to side or tilts his head to one side.**
- **Dog appears to have pain around his ears.** For example, he pulls away or whimpers when you touch his ears.
- **Inflammation or redness of the ear flap or ear canal.** Inflammation of the outer ear canal is called otitis externa, which affects up to 20 percent of dogs
- **Dog scratches or rubs her ears and head against the ground, carpet, furniture, doorways, or other objects.**
- **Presence of scabs or crusty skin on the inner ear flap.**
- **Loss of hair around the ear.**
- **Dog loses her balance or walks in circles.**
- **Hearing loss.**

CAUSES OF EAR INFECTIONS AND OTHER EAR PROBLEMS

Dogs can experience ear infections and other ear problems for a number of reasons. Could one of these reasons be behind your dog's ear problems?

- **Ear mites.** These tiny parasites, *Otodectes cynotis*, can cause intense itching in dogs who are hypersensitive. Dogs can scratch so much it results in an infection and/or trauma to the ear.
- **Foreign objects in the ear.** A dog's ears are perfect hiding places for tiny thorns or "stickers" from grass, foxtails, or wooded areas. If these objects

get into the ear canal, they cause irritation and scratching. It doesn't take long before your dog has an infection. Be sure to check your dog's ears after he comes in from outdoors.

- **Hair growing in the ears.** Some breeds, such as schnauzers, are more likely to have hair growing in their ears, which can become infected.
- **Water in the ears.** If your dog swims or gets frequent baths, water that lodges in the ear can lead to ear infections as well.
- **Allergies, including atopic dermatitis and food allergies.** In fact, ear problems (e.g., scratching, shaking the head) are often the first sign of an allergy, because allergies can alter the environment inside the ear and promote infection.
- **Trauma.** A blow to the head or ears may cause a ruptured eardrum and an accumulation of fluids in the ear canal or the development of a hematoma (blood blister).
- **Hormone changes.** Excessive or deficient levels of some hormones can result in ear problems. For example, low levels of thyroid hormone (a condition called hypothyroidism) and changes in sex hormone levels and hormones produced by the adrenal glands (glucocorticoids) can have an effect on the health of the ears.
- **Ear environment.** Dogs with floppy ears, such as cocker spaniels and other spaniels, golden retrievers, bloodhounds, and poodles, among others, have ears that keep the inner ear flap and ear canal warm and moist, which is a perfect breeding environment for bacteria. An excessive accumulation of earwax and/or oil is another environmental problem in a dog's ears.
- **Hereditary causes.** Rare hereditary diseases affect some dog breeds and have an impact on their

ears. For example, west highland white terriers and shar-peis are susceptible to primary seborrhea (excessively flaky skin), while collies and Shetland sheepdogs may have dermatomyositis (a inherited inflammatory disease of the skin, muscles, and blood vessels).

DIAGNOSING EAR INFECTIONS

Your veterinarian will inspect your dog's ear canal under magnification and look for any foreign objects (including mites, ticks, plant pieces), pus, inflammation, and ingrown hairs. A sample of earwax or discharge from your dog's ears can be examined to identify ear mites, pus, or yeast, or your veterinarian may do a yeast or bacterial culture, especially if your dog has a history of ear infections or the ears are infected and have not responded well to antibiotics in the past.

Because about 20 percent of dogs who experience ear infections and ear inflammation have food allergies, your veterinarian may recommend an elimination diet to identify which foods may be causing this allergic reaction (see also chapter 5, "Atopic Dermatitis").

Ear infections that are not treated properly can lead to chronic pain or even deafness in dogs. That's why it's important to have your dog's ear problems checked by a veterinarian before you treat her at home.

CONVENTIONAL TREATMENT

Regardless of what type of ear problem or ear infection your dog has, the first step is to have the ears cleaned professionally. After that, treatment of ear infections depends on what caused the ear problem and what type of infection developed. For example, if your dog has a bacterial infection, your veterinarian will prescribe antibiotics. It's important to treat bacterial ear infections as quickly as possible, because they can spread to the middle and inner ear and may involve hearing loss. Yeast infections (often caused by *Malassezia pachydermatis)* call for an antifungal medication, since antibiotics do not kill yeast. In both cases, you will also likely be given a prescription for a glucocorticoid such as dexamethasone, which can help reduce ear inflammation.

If, on the other hand, your dog is scratching his ears because of a food allergy, then your veterinarian may recommend allergy shots, antihistamines, and a change in diet (see chapter 5, "Atopic Dermatitis"). A problem with ear mites can be treated with a medication that kills mites, and you may need to administer the drug for several weeks until the mites are gone.

HOME REMEDIES

Make sure you have a diagnosis from your veterinarian before you start any home treatments for your dog. The home remedies explained here are mainly for routine ear washes to help keep your dog's ears free of infections and other problems, and as remedies for yeast infections. Ear infections caused by bacteria typically need antibiotics. However, if you check and clean your dog's ears regularly, use naturally based ear washes as described here, and feed your dog a natural diet, then you can significantly reduce the chances your dog will develop ear infections or other ear problems.

Ear Cleaning at Home

The time you spend cleaning and massaging your dog's ears is time well spent, and chances are your dog will especially love the massage part! To prevent ear infections and other problems, you should clean your dog's ears regularly: once a week for floppy-eared dogs and once a month for dogs with alert ears. If your dog has an ear infection, then ear cleaning should be done three to four times a day when the infection first appears and then reduced as the infection resolves.

Homemade ear washes help maintain the natural environment of the ear, remove excess wax and oil (bacteria thrive in oily, waxy ears), and help prevent disease. A simple vinegar ear wash (see facing page) is generally sufficient for general cleaning, or you can choose an herbal solution for additional benefits. After selecting an ear wash, pour several teaspoons of the solution into your dog's ear. Gently massage the area around the base of the ear for fifteen to thirty seconds, then allow your dog to shake her head to get rid of the excess liquid and any debris in the ear. If the ears are especially dirty, you can repeat this process. Use a soft cloth to remove any extra liquid.

You can use cotton swabs to clean the inside of the ear flap and the area of the ear canal you can see. However, if your dog is not fond of having her ears cleaned and tends to squirm, it's best to forego the cotton swabs to prevent possibly injuring your dog's ears. Cotton swabs should NEVER be used to clean deeper into your dog's ears, even if your dog is well behaved. Use a soft cotton cloth to clean your dog's ears.

Ear Massage

If you think giving your dog an ear massage falls into the category of pampering, you're partially right. However, an ear massage also is an excellent way to improve blood circulation and nerve health in your dog's ears. You might even call ear massage a poor man's acupuncture. The ear has points that correspond to systems throughout the body, and so an ear massage can act as ear (auricular) acupuncture and benefit your dog's entire body.

To give your dog an ear massage, hold the base of one ear with one hand and take the ear flap between the fingers and thumb of your other hand. Gently rub the ear flap in a circular motion starting at the base of the ear and moving toward the tip. This rubbing motion stretches the ear. Your dog should love it!

Diet

It's important to remember that ear infections in dogs are generally the result of a weakened immune system, and one of the best ways to prevent such weakness is to feed your dog a natural diet, described in the first part of this book. If your dog has an ear infection caused by bacteria and your veterinarian has given you a prescription for antibiotics, the medication may eliminate the infection, but it will not benefit your dog's immune system. In fact, prolonged use of antibiotics and other medications, such as steroids, can greatly compromise the ability of your dog's immune system to bounce back. You may want to consider giving your dog probiotics to help restore your dog's bacterial balance if antibiotics are in the picture. (See "Probiotics" on page 136.)

Dogs who experience chronic ear infections may very well have food allergies, so it may be time to try a food elimination diet (see chapter 5, "Atopic Dermatitis"). So once again, feeding your dog a nutritious, toxin-free diet is a key tool in the prevention and management of ear infections.

Vinegar Ear Treatments and Wash

If your dog has a yeast infection in her ears, combine one part apple cider vinegar or white vinegar with one part water. Use an eyedropper to place the mixture into your dog's ears and massage the bases of the ears to disperse the liquid. Wipe out any excess fluid with cotton balls or a soft cloth and allow your dog to shake her head. Treat once or twice daily. This vinegar mixture can also be used as an ear wash once or twice a month to help remove debris and deter bugs.

For bacterial ear infections, combine 3 parts apple cider or white vinegar with 1 part witch hazel. This combination delivers a two-fisted effect: The vinegar changes the pH of the ear canal and the witch hazel has a drying effect and also acts as both an anti-inflammatory and an antiseptic. Use this combination twice a day until your dog's ear infection resolves.

Garlic

Garlic is a natural antibiotic, which makes it a good choice to treat bacterial ear infections. Cathy Alinovi, DVM, offers a garlic ear remedy: Squeeze several cloves of garlic into 3 ounces of olive oil. Add 1 to 2 capsules of vitamin E and let the mixture "brew" for three to four days, then strain through cheesecloth or a fine strainer. Use an eyedropper to apply a few drops into your dog's ear canal twice a day and massage into the ear canal.

An alternative is to combine equal parts of garlic oil and mullein oil. Common mullein (*Verbascum thapsus*) is a plant whose flowers have antimicrobial properties. For every ounce of mullein and garlic oil, add 10 to 20 drops of olive oil. Treat your dog twice a day.

Calendula

Calendula (marigold) has antifungal properties and is also helpful in wound healing. For yeast infections or irritated ears, prepare an ear wash using one teaspoon tincture of calendula along with $\frac{1}{2}$ teaspoon of sea salt and 8 ounces of filtered water. Flush your dog's affected ears once or twice daily until the infection clears.

Green Tea Ear Wash

Green tea is a gentle homemade ear wash you can use regularly to clean your dog's ears. Steep two green tea bags in boiling water for 15 to 20 minutes and allow the tea to cool before using. Flush the ears for routine cleaning.

Other Homemade Remedies

- **Oregon grape** (*Mahonia aquifolium*) has antimicrobial activity against yeast and bacterial infections, and it also can be used to treat ear mites. Apply 1 to 10 drops of Oregon grape tincture in each ear once or twice daily until the infection or the ear mites have disappeared. A few drops of garlic oil can also be added.
- **Hydrogen peroxide** and water, in equal proportions, is a great way to help dissolve excess ear wax in your dog's ears. Apply with an eye dropper or flush the ears.
- **Neem oil solution** can be used to help prevent yeast and bacterial infections after you have cleaned the ears with an ear wash (e.g., vinegar, green tea). Combine the following ingredients and use 10 to 20 drops per ear:
  - ✓ 1 ounce neem oil
  - ✓ $\frac{1}{2}$ ounce olive oil
  - ✓ 1 teaspoon tea tree oil
  - ✓ $\frac{1}{2}$ teaspoon eucalyptus oil

AT-HOME WAYS TO PREVENT EAR INFECTIONS

✓ **Feed your dog a natural diet.** This is the best way to avoid food allergies and to support and maintain a healthy immune system, and thus ward off infections.

(continued)

✓ **Inspect your dog's ears regularly.** Be especially sure to check her ears after she has come back inside from being around grasses or wooded areas.

✓ **Clean your dog's ears regularly.** A slight amount of waxy buildup is normal, but you want to avoid excess accumulation. An effective way to clean your dog's ears involves a two-step process, offered by Dr. Alinovi. First, make a solution comprised of 8 ounces of water plus 1 to 2 drops of mild dish soap. Apply gently inside your dog's ears and massage it into the ear canal. Let your dog shake her head to get rid of the excess water. Then combine 6 ounces of water and 2 ounces of apple cider vinegar. Again massage this mixture into your dog's ear canal and let her shake her head. This ear cleaning method can be used once a week as a preventive step or before starting treatment for an ear infection.

✓ **Prevent water from getting inside your dog's ears.**

✓ **Trim the hairs around and inside your dog's ears regularly.** This will allow more airflow and help prevent moisture buildup.

Chapter 11

Fleas and Ticks

Fleas and ticks: Next to worms (and we discuss those icky creatures later in this book), these annoying and often disease-causing insects are a dog's worst enemies from the creature kingdom. (They aren't too welcome in your home, either!) One reason we tackle fleas and ticks in the same chapter is that along with being the most common external parasites that affect dogs, they also can be treated in similar ways. However, although they have some common characteristics, they are not the same, so we will discuss them separately and then talk about how to eliminate them and make your dog flea-free and tick-free.

FLEAS

Fleas are equal opportunity pests: in fact, the common cat flea (*Ctenocephalides felis*) also makes its home on dogs, biting their skin and causing them to itch and scratch. For some dogs, flea bites are a minor irritation. For dogs who are highly sensitive to flea saliva, however, the itching can be so severe, it causes them to scratch until they lose hair and break the skin, introducing the chance for infection.

It's not enough that fleas bite your dog and make her miserable; they can also transport tapeworms (see chapter 16, worms [Intestinal Parasites]). The best way to prevent a tapeworm infestation is to prevent fleas. The relationship between fleas and tapeworms goes like this: If Blossom the

Boxer/Lab mix has fleas, she will bite at and ingest them. Once she eats fleas that have baby tapeworms, the babies are released from the fleas and attach to the Blossom's intestinal tract, where they suck blood from the intestinal wall and grow into long, segmented worms. Some of the segments contain tapeworm eggs, which then break off and hitch a ride in Blossom's feces. Fleas then feed on the segments and ingest the tapeworm eggs in the segments, and the eggs hatch inside the fleas. That starts the entire cycle all over again.

Does My Dog Have Fleas?

Dogs can scratch themselves for a number of reasons, so you don't need to jump to conclusions just because your dog is scratching. To discover whether fleas are the reason your dog is scratching, look for the telltale signs: black and white specks on your dog skin and fur, and/or seeing the active fleas. The white specks are flea eggs, while black particles are flea poop.

Fleas do not have wings, but they have six legs that they use much to their advantage to both jump and move rapidly through a dog's fur, so it can be difficult to catch them. In fact, fleas can leap as high as four feet, which means the little pests can also jump on you, your furniture, and everything else in your home. If you're starting to itch just thinking about it, just imagine how your dog feels!

On your dog, the most common place to see fleas or evidence of fleas is around the tail and hindquarters and behind the ears. Use a fine-tooth flea comb and run it through your dog's fur or separate the fur with your fingers to find the remnants of fleas or the fleas themselves. You can also comb your dog while he stands on a white sheet to capture the eggs and flea feces. This should give you an idea of the extent of the flea problem.

TICKS

Ticks come in a number of varieties and can be found in nearly every part of the United States, but the two we are most concerned with are the American dog tick and the smaller deer tick. The male dog tick is about the size of a match head, while deer ticks can fit nicely on a pinhead. Female dog ticks (only the females feast on blood) can be recognized by a silver spot behind their head. Depending on where you live, you and your dog may have to deal with one or both of these blood-sucking insects, which are most prevalent during the spring and fall.

Both types of ticks have eight legs and look something like flat spiders; that is, until they begin sucking blood from your dog, and then they look like gray or black bloated bubbles about the size of a plump pea with a head attached to your dog's skin. After the female ticks mate, they have their blood feast and lay their eggs on a dog's skin. It's important to remove ticks as soon as possible, because the females lay their eggs about five to twenty hours after they attach themselves to a dog. Ticks also must be attached to their host for several hours before they can transmit any diseases they may carry, so again, removing them promptly is strongly recommended to help prevent disease.

Another type of tick is the brown dog tick, also known as the kennel tick because it thrives indoors and is usually seen in kennels. However, if you have several dogs and/or your dogs have been in a kennel, look for these insects as well.

Removing Ticks

You should regularly check your dog for ticks, especially if you live in a wooded, grassy, or otherwise rural area or you take your dog for walks in such locations. Although ticks can attach themselves anywhere on a dog's skin, they are usually found between the toes, around the ears, and in the armpits—all places where there is less fur.

If you find a tick on your dog, wear gloves to avoid touching the insect with your skin, because they carry a variety of diseases that affects humans, dogs, and other animals, including Lyme disease (transmitted by deer ticks), Rocky Mountain spotted fever (American dog ticks), and canine ehrlichiosis (brown dog ticks), among others. Use tweezers to remove the tick. These critters can hold on very tight, so if you place a drop of rubbing alcohol or vegetable oil on the tick before you pull it off, this may make removal easier.

If you have discovered the tick before it has buried its head in your dog's skin, then it will be easier to remove. Grasp the tick near your dog's skin where the insect's head is attached and pull straight back; do not twist as you pull, and never break open the bloated tick. Place the tick in a jar of rubbing alcohol until it is dead.

If the tick's head is buried in your dog's skin and you are not successful in getting the tick's head and/or mouth out of the skin, your dog may develop some redness and swelling at the bite site. To help avoid infection, place a small amount of antibiotic ointment on the bite, and the reaction should clear up in two to three days. If the bite gets worse, see your veterinarian.

Ticks transmit disease through their saliva while they are attached and feeding on their host, because the saliva enters the bloodstream. Similar to fleas, the saliva of ticks also can cause your dog to experience an allergic hypersensitive reaction.

CONVENTIONAL TREATMENT

Dozens of OTC and prescription products are available to prevent, control, and treat fleas and ticks. Each product is different: some repel and kill adult fleas and eggs, while others also help eliminate ticks as well. Some are in liquid or gel form and are applied to your dog's skin; others deliver their poisons in a collar, tablets, spray, shampoo/dip, or powder.

The one thing most flea and tick medications have in common is that they are poison, and they can harm your dog if they are not used properly, and in some cases even when they are used as directed. One obvious problem is that dogs lick themselves, and if the poison is on their fur and skin, then they can ingest it. However, there are some natural products on the market that contain some of the ingredients mentioned in the "Home Remedies" section on page 155, which means you can prepare similar treatments yourself.

While dogs can't lick a flea collar, the poisons in these products often cause dogs to lose the hair around their neck and/or develop skin irritations. If you use any OTC or prescription flea and/or tick medication and your dog begins to drool heavily or shake, take him to a veterinarian immediately and bring the flea and tick product with you. And remember: If you do use a commercial flea product, only use ones designated for dogs. Never use a product designed for cats on dogs, and vice versa.

TREATING MORE THAN YOUR DOG FOR FLEAS

Does your dog have fleas? Then your house probably has them too. And you. And other pets in your home. In fact, some veterinarians estimate that for every flea you see on your dog, there are about one hundred more in your house. That's why treating your dog for fleas is not enough, or you and your dog will never get rid of the fleas. So here's what you need to do—and without the use of toxins.

(continued)

✓ **Vacuum your home thoroughly, including the furniture, rugs, and anything covered in fabric.** Throw out the vacuum bag.

✓ **Keep carpets, throw rugs, and anything made of fabric as dry as possible.** Moisture and humidity promote fleas.

✓ **Steam-clean carpets and floors to remove flea larvae.**

✓ **Wash throw rugs and bedding.**

✓ **Treat carpeting with diatomaceous earth (food grade) or a boric acid–based powder.** Sprinkle the product on your carpet, brush it in using a broom, then vacuum. Both diatomaceous earth and boric acid powders are effective against flea larvae but will not harm pets or people, including children.

✓ **Capture fleas using a homemade trap.** Hang a light source over a piece of flypaper or a bowl of soapy water, and the light will attract the fleas to the paper or water.

✓ **Treat your yard and garden.** This may seem like a daunting task, but concentrate on areas your dog goes to often. Fleas breed in shady, moist areas, so clean up wet leaves, pine needles, and debris from under trees, bushes, and decks. A safe, natural way to treat the yard is with microscopic worms called nematodes, which feast on flea larvae and grubs but don't harm your lawn garden, pets, or family. Diatomaceous earth also can be used in your yard. Both of these products should be available at a garden center.

HOME REMEDIES

You don't need to use poisons to prevent or treat fleas and ticks on your dog. Some of the home remedies may already be in your kitchen. In fact, if you are standing near your kitchen sink, you may be looking at one right now: dishwashing detergent. Adding a few drops of mild dishwashing detergent to your dog's bath can kill fleas. Just be sure to rinse your dog off thoroughly to avoid any possible skin reactions.

Use your own judgment: If your dog already has a massive flea infestation and you feel as if you are living in the middle of a flea circus, then your situation may be beyond the home remedies stage. However, for preventive purposes or for mild to moderate problems, these remedies may do the trick. Natural remedies do not have the staying power (nor the toxicity!) of chemicals, so it's necessary to use them daily or every few days, depending on the remedy you choose.

Brewer's Yeast

Fleas reportedly do not like brewer's yeast, and although there are no scientific studies to support its use against fleas in dogs, many pet parents and veterinarians say it works. Add 1 to 3 teaspoons of brewer's yeast (depending on the size of your dog) to your dog's food each day right before flea season is set to begin and throughout the entire time. Brewer's yeast supplements for dogs are also available, and most also contain garlic and other ingredients, such as zinc and biotin.

Another way to use brewer's yeast to fight fleas is to mix 1/4 cup brewer's yeast in 32 ounces of water. Shake well and put in a spray bottle. Spray your dog and work the mixture into his fur.

Citrus

Some research has shown that the main component of citrus peel oil, D-limonene, is deadly to all stages of the cat flea. Flea products often contain citrus extract, but you can make your own at home. Slice an unpeeled orange or two lemons or limes and add the slices to 32 ounces of boiling water. Allow the mixture to steep and cool, then put it in a spray bottle and apply it to your dog. Thoroughly rub it into the fur and skin. Treat once a day or as needed.

Some pet parents swear by a stronger approach: using a freshly squeezed lemon or orange and working the juice directly into their dog's fur. This can make your dog's fur sticky, but that may be small price to pay to discourage fleas. And your dog may love the taste!

Diatomaceous Earth

Diatomaceous earth is a nontoxic substance composed of finely ground skeletal remains of one-celled algae-like plants called diatoms that lived in the water and ended up in chalky deposits of diatomite. The main ingredients in diatomaceous earth are silicon (33 percent) and calcium (19 percent), with much lesser amounts of sodium, magnesium, iron, and trace minerals. I've already mentioned you can treat your house and yard with diatomaceous earth, but it can work wonders for your dog too. Although the powdered substance looks harmless, a microscopic examination will reveal sharp-edged particles that can mean the end of fleas once they pierce the pests and cause them to dehydrate. However, diatomaceous earth is safe for your dog if you use FOOD–GRADE and not gardening/pool-grade products. Even if he licks diatomaceous earth off his fur, food-grade products will not harm him.

Depending on the size of your dog, you need 1 to 6 table-spoons of diatomaceous earth per treatment. Sprinkle a portion of the powder along your dog's spine and rub it into the fur against the way the hair is growing. Apply the remaining powder on other areas of the body, especially the belly, legs, and feet. Try to get the powder distributed throughout the fur, but don't rub it hard into the skin. When applying diatomaceous earth, do it gently and try not to breath in the dust because it can be somewhat irritating for some people and dogs. Once the dust settles, however, it won't be bothersome.

If your dog has lots of fleas, diatomaceous earth works best if you bath your dog first, comb her with a flea comb and let her dry thoroughly before you apply the first treatment. You may need to treat her daily for several days until the fleas begin to disappear. If the flea infestation is mild or moderate, you can apply diatomaceous earth every three to five days.

Garlic

If you search the literature, you won't find scientific studies declaring garlic is an effective preventive or treatment for fleas in dogs. However, many veterinarians will tell you they have pet parents who swear garlic works—and plenty of vets agree. As long as you don't overdo it, garlic may be an effective way to deal with fleas.

Garlic contains allicin and alliin, sulfur compounds that have medicinal properties. If your dog will eat garlic, mince or chop one clove, raw or lightly cooked, for each 10 pounds of your dog's weight and add it to her food each day.

Neem

Neem seed extract and neem oil are derived from the neem tree, or *Azadirachta indica*. The oil, leaves, and bark of the neem tree have been valued for thousands of years in India, and they are used around the world today for various purposes, including as a natural insect repellent. Neem extract and oil are common ingredients in flea shampoo for dogs, and you can make your own by adding a few drops of neem to a flea dip or to your dog's shampoo if it does not contain neem. Scientific studies back up the use of neem seed extract as effective against fleas, ticks, and mites.

Other Home Remedies

- **Lavender oil.** A mixture of lavender oil and sweet almond oil will not kill fleas, but it can repel them. Combine 10 drops of lavender oil and 5 drops to 10 ml of sweet almond oil in a spray bottle, shake well, and spritz your dog. Avoid her face and ears.
- **Rose geranium oil.** The essential oil of rose geranium is derived from the leaves of the *Pelargonium graveolens* plant, one of the scented geraniums. This oil reportedly can repel ticks (and possibly fleas) when applied to your skin or to your dog. Some commercial tick repellent products contain rose geranium oil. To use rose geranium oil for your dog, place a few drops on your dog's collar. If a tick has already attached itself to your dog, place a drop of rose geranium oil directly onto the tick, and the critter should drop off shortly.
- **Rosemary.** The herb rosemary can repel fleas on your dog in two ways. One, grind fresh rosemary leaves into a powder and sprinkle them where your dog sleeps. Two, steep ½ cup of fresh rosemary leaves in boiling water for thirty minutes, then add to 1 gallon of warm water. Soak your dog with this mixture—do not dilute it further. Let your dog dry naturally. She will smell nice, and because rose-

mary is an anti-inflammatory, it can help relieve itching too.

- **Vinegar.** Make those pesky fleas flee with apple cider vinegar. Make sure you use this remedy outdoors, because the fleas will jump off your dog. Combine 2 parts apple cider vinegar (white will do if you don't have apple cider) with 1 part water in a spray bottle. Soak your dog's fur and then comb thoroughly. Repeat every three to four days.

Chapter 12

Kidney Problems

Kidney problems in dogs can be sneaky. Your dog, Frieda, seems to be perfectly fine: Her appetite is good, she loves her walks, and she's eliminating in all the right places. Then you notice Frieda is drinking more water than usual, but you figure it may be the warmer weather, until she starts asking to go outside to pee more than she used to. *Okay,* you think, *it makes sense for her to pee more if she's drinking more,* so although your radar has been tweaked, it doesn't go off until Frieda walks away from her breakfast—her favorite recipe, too—and then her dinner. Now you're getting alarmed, and when you take her to the veterinarian the next day and the tests are done, the diagnosis shocks you. Kidney disease! How could that happen?

Kidney disease (also referred to as renal disease or kidney failure) is common in dogs, especially as they approach their senior years. However, not every case of kidney disease or kidney failure is associated with aging, so kidney problems can affect a dogs at any time during her lifetime.

Let's clear up the term "kidney failure" right from the start, because it is often used by veterinarians and in the literature. "Kidney failure" suggests that the kidneys have stopped working and no longer produce urine. That is not true. The definition of kidney failure is the inability of the kidneys to remove waste materials from the blood. It means the kidneys are overworked or even damaged (i.e., severe chronic renal failure). However, dogs with kidney failure still produce urine, and in fact often make more than normal.

To better understand why it's important for you to know more about kidney disease, you first should know a little more about kidneys.

WHY KIDNEYS ARE IMPORTANT

The kidneys are a pair of small organs that are made up of thousands of minute funnels, called nephrons, that filter the blood and balance fluid levels in the body. Other functions of the kidneys include producing hormones involved in the production of red blood cells; regulating levels of calcium, phosphorus, and magnesium; and keeping blood pressure within normal limits.

Dogs, like their pet parents, have lots of extra nephrons, which is both good and bad: good because the extras can fill in when nephrons become damaged and can't function any longer; bad because as the number of functioning nephrons declines, the kidneys lose their ability to filter out toxins and maintain healthy fluid balance. When nephron levels drop below 25 percent, symptoms of kidney disease typically appear. Therefore kidney disease can be progressing in your dog before you know about it unless you have urine and blood tests conducted regularly to identify any changes.

As the number of functioning nephrons declines, the kidneys lose their ability to filter out toxins and maintain healthy fluid balance. When nephron levels drop below 25 percent, symptoms of kidney disease become evident. Although chronic kidney failure cannot be reversed or cured, there are effective ways to treat and manage the symptoms and slow disease progression.

DOES MY DOG HAVE KIDNEY DISEASE?

Kidney disease can be insidious because the early stages of disease are characterized by symptoms that are easy to miss or that can be associated with aging. If your dog has any of the following symptoms, it may indicate kidney disease. They include:

- drinking an excessive amount of water
- frequent urination (easy to miss if your dog stays outside a great deal of the time)
- urine that is pale to nearly clear in color and with hardly any odor
- urine leakage (seen more often in females)
- weight loss
- loss of appetite
- vomiting
- chemical smell to the breath
- lethargy or depression
- mouth ulcers
- pale gums
- muscle weakness.

As in the case of Frieda in the opening of this chapter, it is easy to miss the possibility of kidney disease until a dog suddenly stops eating. That's when pet parents often think back and realize there were some indications of kidney disease for a while, but nothing seemingly alarming.

As a dog's kidney function fails, her blood and tissues accumulate chemical wastes, such as ammonia, nitrogen, and acids. This is called uremia, and a veterinarian can determine the severity of uremia by conducting a chemistry panel. (See "Diagnosing Kidney Disease" on page 164.). If your dog has uremia, you will notice weight loss, depression, a dry haircoat, an ammonia-like smell to her breath, a brownish tongue, and mouth ulcers. Diarrhea, vomiting, and gastrointestinal bleeding may also occur. The end stage of kidney failure involves coma and death.

Although dogs of any breed can get kidney disease or experience kidney failure, certain breeds are at greater risk, including bull terriers, cairn terriers, English cocker spaniels, German shepherds, and Samoyeds.

TYPES AND CAUSES OF KIDNEY DISEASE

Kidney disease appears in two main forms: acute or chronic. Acute disease (acute kidney failure) comes on suddenly and can be very serious and life-threatening. Causes of acute kidney failure can include any of the following:

- **Poisoning, which is a common cause of acute kidney failure.** The poisons most frequently ingested by dogs are rat poison (contains calciferol) and antifreeze (ethylene glycol, which has a sweet taste). Just one big lick (about 1 teaspoon) of an ethylene glycol–based antifreeze, for example, can completely shut down a dog's kidneys. If vomiting is induced immediately and the dog is treated by a veterinarian, the dog has a chance of survival. Dogs who ingest calciferol experience an accumulation of calcium in the body that damages the kidneys.
- **Ruptured bladder or urethra.** This is usually associated with an accident such as getting hit by a car
- **Congestive heart failure.** This reduces blood flow to the kidneys
- **Blockage of the urinary tract caused by a stone.**
- **Lyme disease, which is transmitted by ticks.**
- **Diabetes.**
- **Leptospirosis, a bacterial disease that can damage the kidneys.** Adult dogs males and large-breed

dogs seem to be more susceptible to contracting leptospirosis, although any dog can develop the infection, especially if he is exposed to rodents, which carry the bacteria.
- **Genetic factors.**

The biggest obstacle to beating acute kidney disease is if the dog can survive the damage done to his kidneys from going into shock. Acute kidney failure can be reversed if a dog receives the right treatment in a timely manner and gets past the shock stage.

Chronic kidney disease is the slow, "silent" type, because it usually comes on gradually with advancing age or as the result of an inherited or congenital condition, the signs of which are less specific. Another cause of chronic kidney failure that many pet parents don't realize is dental disease: bacteria that invade your dog's mouth, especially in the advanced stages of gum disease (periodontitis; see chapter 7, "Dental Disease"), can get into your dog's bloodstream and travel to various organs, including the kidneys.

You can't reverse aging nor congenital conditions, nor can you reverse chronic kidney disease, but you can significantly slow its progress. Home remedies can be an important part of this strategy.

DIAGNOSING KIDNEY DISEASE

Because kidney disease can be a silent malady, veterinarians often recommend that dogs have their first baseline urine and blood test at age three if they are large and around age five if they are small. The values will tell your veterinarian what normal levels are for your dog and subsequent tests (recommended yearly) can identify any changes that indicate kidney disease. If you are thinking, *This sounds expen-*

sive, you are right, but it is important to at least have your dog's baseline values on record. If you provide your dog with a wholesome diet as discussed in earlier chapters, then you will have an excellent start in preventing or limiting damage from the most common type of kidney problem, chronic kidney disease associated with advancing age.

Veterinarians use a number of tests to help identify and diagnose kidney disease, its severity, and its causes:

- **Chemistry panel.** A chemistry panel is a group of chemistry tests conducted on blood samples to identify certain values. For kidney disease in dogs, typical values are blood urea nitrogen (BUN), creatinine, phosphorus, and potassium. BUN is a by-product of protein metabolism. If a dog's kidneys are not working properly, BUN builds up in the blood, as does creatinine. Phosphorus levels rise in kidney disease because less of the mineral is excreted into the urine by the kidneys. Potassium levels rise when kidneys fail, resulting in a condition called hyperkalemia, which causes fatigue, nausea, and a slow heartbeat.
- **Urinalysis.** This involves multiple tests performed on a urine sample. Veterinarians look for a concentration of urine (urine specific gravity) with a range of 1.008 to 1.015, indicating possible kidney disease. They also look for high levels of protein and analyze any sediment in the urine, which may indicate the cause of the kidney problem.
- **Complete blood count.** A complete blood count can identify anemia, a low red blood cell level, which is common in cases of kidney failure. Anemia can cause fatigue and weakness.
- **X-rays.** Your veterinarian may take X-rays to identify the size and shape of your dog's kidneys. Small

kidneys are more common in dogs who have chronic kidney disease, while large kidneys may have an acute kidney problem or cancer.

- **Ultrasound.** Infrequently, veterinarians suggest an ultrasound to look for changes in a dog's kidney density. If a biopsy is taken during an ultrasound, it may help identify the cause of a dog's kidney disease.

CONVENTIONAL TREATMENT

Regardless of whether your dog's kidney problems are acute or chronic, prompt treatment is important. Obviously, "prompt" treatment for kidney failure associated with poisoning is different from that for chronic kidney problems associate with aging. Medical treatment of both acute and chronic kidney disease is somewhat similar and has the same purpose in both cases: to support kidney function until the organ is able to return to normal or reasonable operation on its own.

In most cases, dogs who experience acute kidney failure, even when treated immediately, suffer some degree of kidney damage. This means the dogs will need permanent changes in their diet and perhaps additional medical care, such as occasional subcutaneous fluids (sub-Q, which pet parents can often learn to do at home) to prevent dehydration and restore electrolyte levels, or dialysis. Some dogs will need medications as well, such as antihypertensives to lower blood pressure or erythropoietin to stimulate the production of red blood cells, which will increase the amount of oxygen in the tissues. Dogs who have chronic kidney failure will need disease management for the rest of their lives. Part of any dog's treatment program will include periodic monitoring of the blood to follow changes in kidney function.

Dietary changes will include restricted salt intake to help

prevent high blood pressure and ascites (an accumulation of fluid in the abdominal cavity) and potassium to prevent heart problems. Phosphorus intake also should be limited, because the kidneys help regulate phosphorus levels in the bloodstream. When kidney function is impaired, phosphorus levels can build up, which in turn lowers calcium levels in the blood and contributes to bone disease. Generally, phosphorus is highest in foods high in protein, but some meats, dairy products, beans, and fish are lower in phosphorus than others. Veterinarians can prescribe medications to lower phosphorus levels, but dietary changes are still necessary.

Some veterinarians believe protein is a problem for dogs who have kidney failure. However, studies have shown that dogs with renal failure who are put on a low-protein diet not only do not get better, they decline. Generally it is best to customize the protein content of the diet for each dog who has kidney failure and to avoid commercially processed foods. (See "Home Remedies" on page 168.)

Dialysis is a treatment option frequently used for dogs with acute kidney failure, especially in cases of antifreeze or other poisoning, and is available in two forms. Peritoneal dialysis is a technique in which a catheter is placed into the dog's abdomen to deliver special fluids that bathe the tissues and absorb toxins. The fluid then is removed through the catheter. Hemodialysis is another type of dialysis, and this one circulates the dog's blood through a machine that acts like the kidneys and filters out the toxins. Hemodialysis is a costly procedure and less available.

Dogs with terminal kidney failure can be considered for a kidney transplant. After the transplant, these dogs require drugs to prevent organ rejection and careful monitoring to minimize side effects associated with these medications.

When all is said and done, prompt treatment and a change in lifestyle—specifically diet—can allow many dogs with kidney problems to live a long, normal life.

HOW TO PREVENT KIDNEY DISEASE

There are some steps you can take to help prevent kidney disease:

- Lock up and /or remove any poisons or toxins that your dog could access, such as antifreeze, pesticides, and rat poison.
- Do not keep any dangerous chemicals in the yard or other areas where your dog may spend time.
- Keep your dog on a nutritious, whole foods diet.
- Never give your dog medications without first consulting with your veterinarian.
- Maintain good oral hygiene, including daily tooth brushing (see chapter 7, "Dental Disease").

HOME REMEDIES

Home remedies for dogs who have kidney disease or kidney failure involve dietary changes, which you can support with natural supplements. Here are some suggestions on how to manage kidney failure in your dog using home remedies:

Diet

According to Dr. Pitcairn in his book *Dr. Pitcairn's Complete Guide to Natural Health for Dogs and Cats,* the preservatives, artificial flavorings and artificial colorings that are added to foods—as well as the contaminants prevalent in the air, water, and soil—are "directly stressful to the kidneys and probably play a role in the development of the condition [kidney failure]."

Feeding your dog low-quality protein makes her kidneys

work harder, while high-quality protein allows her kidneys to process and eliminate more waste products, which in turn helps preserve kidney function. Diets for dogs that have kidney failure control the amount of protein, phosphorus, salt, potassium, magnesium, and B vitamins. When you introduce the new food to your dog, do it gradually over one to two weeks so she will be more likely to accept it and it is less stressful to the kidneys.

Here are several homemade recipes for dogs who have kidney failure. Also see the list of foods that are low in phosphorus and high in potassium for dogs with kidney failure. Consult your veterinarian before trying any new diet for kidney failure for your dog.

Spuds and Egg

1 large egg, hard boiled
1 cup mashed white potato with skin
1 cup mashed sweet potato with skin
$1/2$ cup green peas, cooked
Calcium supplement
Multivitamin/mineral supplement (1 per day)

Chop up the hard-boiled egg and mix it with the other ingredients. You may choose to give the supplements separately. This recipe is sufficient for one day for a 40- to 50-pound dog, divided into 2 to 3 servings.

Chicken and Veggies

2 cups cooked chicken breast, cubed
2 cups cooked sweet potato with skin, cubed
2 cups lightly steamed broccoli, carrots, and/or cabbage
$1/4$ cup no-salt chicken broth
Calcium supplement
Multivitamin/mineral supplement

Combine all ingredients, although you may give the supplements separately. This is enough for a 40- to 50-pound dog for two to four days, divided into 2 to 3 servings daily.

Beans and Rice

2 cups cooked brown rice
1 cup cooked pinto beans
2 eggs, hard boiled
$1/2$ cup cooked chicken breast
2 cups lightly cooked sliced carrots and/or chopped
   broccoli
Calcium and multivitamin/mineral supplements

Combine all ingredients. You can give the supplements separately. This recipe is sufficient for one 40- to 50-pound dog for two to three days fed in divided servings.

SAFE FOODS FOR DOGS WITH KIDNEY FAILURE

Note: All foods contain phosphorus, so it's impossible to avoid it completely. Therefore, focus on foods low in phosphorus.
Low phosphorus: All fruits and vegetables, barley, eggs, rice, couscous, rice noodles, refined pasta
Moderate phosphorus (use in limited amounts): Beans, beef, chicken, canned tuna (in water), rockfish, sea bass, turkey
High potassium: Beans (some varieties), broccoli, cabbage, cantaloupe, carrots, halibut, lentils, mushrooms, pumpkin, rice bran, spinach, sweet potatoes, white potatoes, yogurt

Omega-3 Fatty Acids

Omega-3 fatty acids are fats that are essential for health but which must be obtained from the diet, since they cannot be manufactured by the body. The main source of omega-3s are fish and fish oil, which provide two primary omega-3s, EPA (eicosapentaenoic acid) and DHA (docosahexaenoic acid). In several clinical trials with dogs, omega-3 fatty acids from marine fish oil were effective in slowing the progression of kidney disease. In research funded by the National Institute of Diabetes and Digestive and Kidney Diseases, it's been reported that omega-3 fatty acids may reduce kidney damage in people with type 1 diabetes. Other research shows that omega-3s reduce blood pressure, heart rate, and triglycerides in people with chronic kidney disease.

Consult your veterinarian about the most beneficial dose of omega-3 fatty acids for your dog. Be sure you give your dog a supplement that contains both EPA and DHA from marine fish oil.

Vitamin E

If you give your dog omega-3 fatty acids, then it is also suggested you supplement with vitamin E, since these two nutrients have a synergistic relationship. The suggested dose of vitamin E is 50 IU for dogs who weigh less than 25 pounds, 100 IUs for dogs who weigh 25 to 60 pounds, and 200 IUs for dogs who weigh more than 60 pounds, given at least two times per week.

Vitamin B Complex

Dogs with kidney failure are not able to properly recycle and retain the water-soluble B vitamins, therefore a vitamin

B–complex supplement is suggested. Although the supplement does not specifically help kidney function, it does help restore necessary levels of B vitamins that dogs with kidney failure lose because they drink more water and urinate more and it may help boost energy level. One suggestion is to give your dog a vitamin B-50 supplement, which provides 50 mg each of B_1, B_2, B_6, B_{12}, biotin, and folic acid.

Vitamin C

Like the B family of vitamins, vitamin C is a water-soluble nutrient that is easily flushed out of the body during excess urination. Even though dogs can make their own vitamin C, dog can lose much of it if they have kidney failure, which is why a vitamin C supplement is recommended. The suggested form is ascorbic acid, because it does not expose your dog to extra calcium, magnesium, or sodium as would some other forms of vitamin C (e.g., calcium ascorbate and sodium ascorbate). Suggested dosing is 100 mg twice a day for dogs weighing 5 to 25 pounds, 250 mg twice daily for dogs weighing 25 to 50 pounds, 500 mg twice daily for large dogs weighing 50 to 75 pounds, and 1,000 mg twice daily for larger dogs. If your dog experiences some diarrhea when taking vitamin C, reduce the dose.

Other Home Remedies

- **Alfalfa.** Alfalfa (*Medicago sativa*) is a supplement frequently used to help strengthen kidney function, although the scientific studies are not supportive. The suggested dose is one tablet per 30 pounds of body weight given once daily added to the dog's food.
- **Baking soda.** Adding a pinch of baking soda (also known as sodium bicarbonate) to your dog's food at every meal may be beneficial. Dogs with kidney

failure pee a lot, and the excessive urination removes bicarbonate ions from the kidneys, which they need to function optimally. Adding baking soda helps replenish the lost sodium bicarbonate.

Chapter 13

Obesity

Chubby puppies are cute, but when chubby puppies become overweight or obese adult dogs, it is a health issue. Obesity is not just a people problem. According to the Association for Pet Obesity Prevention (APOP), which is composed of dedicated veterinarians and veterinary healthcare personnel, an estimated 55.6 percent of the 77.5 million dogs (43 million) in the United States are overweight or obese.

It's no surprise that dogs are overweight for basically the same reasons people are: They consume too many calories, eat between meals, fail to reduce calorie intake as they get older and their metabolism slows, and don't get enough exercise. Each of these reasons is under your control, so you can begin now to take steps to either prevent obesity or help your dog drop those extra pounds.

IS MY DOG TOO FAT?

"Do I look fat in this collar?" "Does this harness make my hips look big?" If your dog could talk, she might ask you these questions if she is carrying around excess pounds. As your dog's health advocate, it is your responsibility to ensure he is not overweight or obese and your responsibility to help him achieve a healthy weight. Yet that's only possible if you take this critical first step: Accept that your dog has a weight problem. Denial by pet parents that their dog is overweight is one of the biggest barriers to successful weight loss for dogs.

You can tell when you've gained weight: That dress and pair of favorite jeans don't fit anymore. But pet parents are not always good at identifying when their dog is too fat. The traditional way to determine your dog's body condition is by look and feel. When standing above your dog and looking down, you should be able to see a well-defined narrowing (a "waistline") below the rib cage and above the hips. The other test is to place your hands on your dog's rib cage, and you should be able to feel the individual ribs without pressing hard. If you cannot feel the individual ribs and your dog has no waistline, then he or she is carrying too much fat.

Some dog breeds naturally tend to be a bit thicker in the waistline than others, including basset hounds, beagles, cairn terriers, cocker spaniels, collies, dachshunds, Labrador retrievers, and Shetland sheepdogs. These dogs will have less of a well-defined waistline. For these dogs, and for any dog for that matter, there is another way to help determine if your dog is too fat.

WILL SPAYING/NEUTERING MAKE MY DOG FAT?

Some people worry that spaying and neutering dogs will make them fat. Yes, some altered dogs do gain weight, but weight gain is the result of a combination of factors: insufficient exercise, eating too many calories, slowed metabolic rate, and hormonal changes. Attention to diet and exercise typically prevents weight gain after a dog has been spayed or neutered.

The Association for Pet Obesity Prevention (APOP) has developed an online pet weight translator (http://www.peto besityprevention.com/pet-weight-translator/) that can help you determine if your dog is overweight in terms that are easy to understand. That is, APOP developed weight equivalent charts so a pet parent can determine how much her pet weighs compared to an average adult human man or woman.

For example, the average healthy weight for a Yorkie is 6 to 8 pounds. A 12-pound Yorkie would be 50 percent overweight and be comparable to an average woman (five feet four inches) weighing 218 pounds. A female golden retriever should weigh 55 to 65 pounds. However, one that tips the scales at 84 pounds is 29 percent overweight and is the equivalent of a five-foot-four-inch woman who weighs 187 pounds.

CAUSES OF OBESITY IN DOGS

The causes of overweight and obesity in dogs are similar to those in people, yet remember you are your dog's health advocate, so you have a great deal of control over whether Sparky eats a high-fat diet or Cleopatra is a couch potato.

- **Insufficient exercise.** It's not rocket science: Physical activity burns calories, and if your dog gets more exercise, he'll use more calories. It's also important for dogs to be physically active because it reduces their levels of stress and boredom, and tense, bored dogs tend to eat more—just like some people do!
- **Poor-quality food.** Many commercial dog foods and treats are high in fat, grains, and sugar, not to mention the preservatives and other artificial ingredients. Even if you choose a high-quality commercial food, a sedentary or moderately active dog can gain weight if he is eating a high-energy dog food. As with people, calories do count!
- **Hypothyroidism.** Infrequently, dogs can develop hypothyroidism, a condition in which the thyroid gland dysfunctions and does not produce enough of

the hormones needed to regulate metabolism. It occurs most often in middle-age dogs of medium and large breeds, but it can develop in any dog of any age or size. The breeds most often affected are Airedale terriers, cocker spaniels, dachshunds, Doberman pinschers, golden retrievers, greyhounds, Irish setters, Labrador retrievers, and Shetland sheepdogs. Dogs with hypothyroidism typically put on weight quickly and experience poor hair regrowth and/or hair loss.

- **Age.** Obesity is most likely to develop in dogs between the ages of two and six years. It's best to nip it in the bud so it doesn't follow your dog into his later years and lead to other health issues, such as osteoarthritis, heart disease, and diabetes, for example.

FAT DOGS AND HEALTH RISKS

Similar to their two-legged pet parents, dogs who are overweight or obese are at increased risk for a number of serious health problems. You should also be aware that obesity in certain breeds presents additional problems. Here are examples of health challenges associated with canine obesity and some of the specific breeds at greater risk. Of course, mixed-breed dogs can be prone to these risks as well.

- **Diabetes.** This is one of the most common complications of overweight and obese dogs (see chapter 8, "Diabetes").
- **Bone, joint, and ligament problems.** The most common health issue in this category is arthritis (see Chapter 4, "Arthritis"). Being overweight can not only contribute to the development of arthritis but also make it worse once it occurs. One breed

susceptible to bone problems associated with obesity is the dachshund. Dachshunds are prone to developing a slipped disk (intervertebral disk disease), and being overweight increases the likelihood they will develop this often debilitating condition. If a slipped disk does occur, the extra weight will make it harder for the dog to recover. Overweight dogs are also more likely to damage their anterior cruciate ligament (ACL), which is located in the knee area. If ACL damage occurs, the knee will be unstable and the dog will be reluctant to use it.

- **High blood pressure.** Just like people, overweight dogs tend to have high blood pressure, since the heart has to work harder to pump blood to the greater amount of tissues.
- **Heart disease.** Excess weight causes the heart to work harder, and this can lead to congestive heart failure.
- **Breathing problems.** Excess fat in the chest and/or diaphragm can restrict a dog's ability to breathe properly, especially breeds that are prone to breathing problems, such as the boxer, bulldog, Chihuahua, Pekingese, pug, and shih tzu.
- **Heat intolerance.** Overweight dogs can easily become overheated during the high temperatures of summer.
- **Impaired liver function.** The liver stores fat, and overweight dogs can accumulate too much fat in the liver (hepatic lipidosis), which can result in a decrease in liver function.
- **Cancer.** Although the reason is not known, there is an increased risk of developing certain types of cancer among obese dogs, including cancer of the urinary bladder and mammary tumors.
- **Reduced immune function.** Obesity in dogs reduces the ability of the immune system to resist

bacterial and viral infections, especially canine distemper and salmonella infections.
- **Decreased quality of life and lifespan.** Overweight dogs die at a younger age than do dogs who stay at a healthy weight. Given the many health problems that can plague an obese dog, it's no surprise that quality of life is affected. Overweight dogs may be in pain, overheated, or uncomfortable, all of which can make them irritable, anxious, or even aggressive.

CONVENTIONAL TREATMENT

Because there are certain medical conditions that can cause dogs to be obese, as well as conditions that can have an effect on how a weight-loss program should be pursued, your veterinarian should examine your dog before you start any type of diet and exercise plan. You and your veterinarian or certified veterinary nutritionist also should discuss how much weight your dog needs to lose and decide upon a safe, realistic goal for that loss, typically 1 to 2 percent of your dog's body weight per week. Therefore, if Napoleon weighs 80 pounds and the goal is 70 pounds, it will take about seven to fourteen weeks for Napoleon to show off his new figure. Once Napoleon reaches his goal, however, the trick is to keep it off. You are in charge: Your efforts will help keep the weight off your dog. That means regular weighing sessions to make sure the weight is not creeping back on while you gradually increase your dog's food intake from the weight-loss level. You can either slightly increase the foods you were using as part of the weight-loss program or switch to another diet that is less limited. However, you may risk having your dog regain the weight if you add too many calories and/or fat and you don't continue with a regular exercise program.

If you choose a commercial dog food, look for specially formulated weight-loss diets that are limited in fat and calories but that are higher than adult maintenance diets in protein and micronutrients. (See the appendix for sources of high-quality dietary formulations.) Unfortunately, many prescription weight-loss dog foods are high in carbohydrates and low in fat and protein. The best way for your dog to lose weight is to consume a diet with balanced high-quality protein and carbohydrates, because high-quality protein will help minimize the amount of lean muscle lost as the pounds drop off.

Doggie Diet Pills

Believe it or not, there is a diet drug for dogs. In January 2007, the Food and Drug Administration approved Slendrol (generic name dirlotapide), made by Pfizer Animal Health. Slendrol suppresses a dog's appetite and blocks the absorption of fat. This drug is the first for treatment of obesity in dogs and may be prescribed by veterinarians for dogs who are not successful in losing weight with diet and exercise (sound familiar?). Dirlotapide should not be used by dogs who are on corticosteroid therapy or those who have liver disease. Vomiting is the most common side effect, although some dogs also experience diarrhea, loss of appetite, and lethargy. Any dog who has these side effects for more than two days should be reevaluated by a veterinarian.

WARNING: NEVER give your dog diet pills, prescription or over-the-counter, that are designed for humans.

HOME HEALTHY TIPS TO HELP YOUR DOG LOSE WEIGHT

✓ **Make eating fun.** Put your dog's meals in a food-dispensing toy. This will make your dog work for his dinner and make the experience more enjoyable. Occasionally you can also freeze his food (you may need to add some moisture to some recipes, such as a small amount of nonfat plain yogurt) and put it in the toy.

✓ **Exercise more.** Allowing your obese dog to play in the backyard by herself is not sufficient: Dogs need supervised or managed exercise. That means it's time to take longer walks, have more play sessions, and perhaps ramp up the vigorousness of the exercise. A word of caution, however: Do not start a new, more intensive exercise program without first consulting your veterinarian. An increase in exercise and activity should be done gradually so your dog's heart, muscles, and respiratory system are not overly stressed. Do not take your overweight dog on a two-mile run, for example; start with a brisk half-mile walk every day for a week, then increase it to a mile, then two, and then perhaps introduce a short jog several times a week. Swimming is a wonderful exercise for dogs, especially those who have arthritis.

✓ **Be strong.** Yes, it's hard to resist those big brown sad eyes that seem to bore right through you and say "I'm starving!" but you can do it. This rule applies to your kids as well: No sneaking food to the dog! Keep low-calorie treats handy to deal with those pleading eyes: cut raw carrots, raw green beans, unbuttered popcorn, apple slices.

✓ **Check fat content.** If you are still feeding your dog commercial dog food, look for foods that contain high-quality protein and carbohydrates and low fat. The average fat content (dry-matter basis) for dry dog food is 16 percent, while a low-fat alternative should contain no more than 10 percent. The average fat content of wet dog food (dry-matter basis) is 23 percent, while a low-fat food should contain less than 15 percent. (See "Deciphering Dog Food Ingredients" on page 38.) If you prepare your own homemade dog food, you can better regulate the fat, protein, and carbohydrate content and quality.

✓ **Introduce new treats.** Treats are synonymous with food, but you can treat your dog with something other than calories. An extra walk about the block is a treat and keeps your dog's focus away from food. New toys are treats as well, as is being groomed. The added attention you give your dog is better than any biscuit!

HOME REMEDIES

The home remedies to fight dog obesity address diet and nutrition on a personal level: You choose and control the ingredients and nutrients your dog will consume, making sure she gets nutritious meals that are low in fat and bursting with high-quality protein and carbohydrates (especially fiber) while tasting great as well. In addition, there are some natural supplements that can make the weight loss and management a little easier.

Low-Fat Ingredients

When it comes to fat content of dog food, the general rule most veterinarians follow is:

- A diet containing less than 10 percent fat on a dry matter basis (which translates into less than 17 percent of calories from fat) is considered low fat.
- A diet containing 10 percent to 15 percent fat (17 percent to 23 percent of calories) is defined as moderate fat.

- A diet containing more than 20 percent fat is high fat.

To prepare a low-fat homemade meal for your overweight or obese dog, a general guideline to follow is 50 percent high-quality carbohydrates and 50 percent low-fat protein sources. The carbohydrates should provide an excellent to very good amount of fiber and nutrients while being low-fat at the same time. Candidates in this category include brown rice, oatmeal, barley, sweet potatoes, winter squash, pumpkin, whole-grain pasta, broccoli, summer squash, green beans, and carrots.

Now for protein, which can include both animal and non-animal sources:

- ✓ Chicken breast and turkey breast (skinless) are low in fat, although other parts can be included if you remove any visible fat.
- ✓ Ground beef is available in different grades, but be sure to cook off the fat and remove it.
- ✓ Fish, especially cold water fatty fish (e.g., salmon, tuna, sardines, mackerel) are low fat and provide excellent amounts of omega-3 fatty acids.
- ✓ Liver and kidney can be included but in small amounts: no more than 1 ounce of organ meat per pound of food.
- ✓ Nonfat or low-fat dairy such as farmer cheese, plain yogurt, and kefir.
- ✓ Eggs are an excellent protein source, but limit the number of yolks you include because they are high in fat (5 grams per yolk).
- ✓ Non-animal protein sources include well-cooked legumes (pinto beans, lentils, split peas), tofu, tempeh, and textured vegetable protein (TVP).

Meats should be cooked at least enough to kill bacteria, and fattier ground beef can be boiled to release the fat, which should be skimmed off while cooking. Grains, beans, and vegetables should be cooked for optimal digestion and nutritional value. Small amounts of fruit (e.g., apple, banana, blueberries, and melon) are good as treats, but avoid avocadoes, which are high in fat.

Low-Fat Recipes

Turkey Bake

3 cups ground turkey (Chicken is okay too.)
2 egg whites
$1\frac{1}{2}$ cups oatmeal
$\frac{1}{2}$ cup grated carrots
$\frac{1}{2}$ cup finely chopped broccoli
$\frac{1}{2}$ cup farmer cheese

Preheat the oven to 350 degrees. Use spray-on oil to grease a 9×13 inch baking pan. Combine all the ingredients for the turkey bake in a bowl and mix well. Press into the baking dish and bake for 35 minutes. Cut into appropriate portions for the size of your dog. Remember that dogs fed a homemade diet need added calcium: 30 mg calcium per pound of body weight daily is recommended. (See "Calcium" on page 26.)

Vegetable and Chicken Delight

$\frac{1}{2}$ lb ground chicken or turkey, cooked
2 cups uncreamed cottage cheese (You can use farmer cheese.)
3 cups lightly cooked grated carrots, shredded cabbage, chopped broccoli or cauliflower (any one or more to make 3 cups)
3 cups plain puréed pumpkin or plain mashed sweet potato

2 cups cooked peas (canned is okay, but no salt),
cooked lentils, or cooked pinto, black, navy,
or white beans, mashed
1 cup rice bran
2 doses of multivitamin/mineral for dogs

Mix all the ingredients together and store the food, covered, in the refrigerator for no more than three days. If your dog is not used to eating vegetables, you might prepare the recipe using half the amount of pumpkin, etc., and gradually increase the amount if your dog responds well to the food. Feed the amount appropriate for your size dog.

Low-Fat Treats

Your dog can still have treats, even if she is on a weight-loss program. Some low-fat treats include lightly cooked carrot sticks or green beans, apple slices, rice cakes, pieces of melon, popcorn (no butter or salt), and banana slices. Avoid commercial dehydrated meat treats, many of which come from China and have been linked to kidney problems. You can make your own dehydrated treats in a food dryer: Try sweet potato slices, thin slices of low-fat meat, dried green beans, mushrooms, apple slices, banana slices. A sprinkling of garlic powder or anise on the meat or vegetables before drying makes them extra tasty.

DHEA

DHEA (dehydroepiandrosterone) is a hormone produced by the adrenal gland in people and other mammals, including dogs. A number of studies in dogs show that supplementation with DHEA can help obese canines lose body weight and body fat. For example, at the University of Wisconsin, where a number of studies have been conducted, researchers used DHEA supplementation and a low-energy (low-calorie), high-fiber diet with obese dogs. Compared with obese dogs who were give just the low-energy, high-fiber diet, those who took DHEA lost significantly more weight, lost weight faster, and also had a reduction in their cholesterol levels.

In another study at the same university, obese dogs were given DHEA for three months at an increasing dose of 30 to 75 mg/kg per day. Sixty-eight percent of the obese dogs lost 3 percent of their total body weight per month without following a low-energy diet. They also had a significant reduction in their cholesterol levels.

Consult your veterinarian before giving your dog DHEA to help with weight loss. He or she will determine the optimal dose you can give your dog at home.

L-Carnitine

This amino acid is synthesized in the kidneys and liver from two other amino acids, lysine and methionine, with the help of vitamin C. L-carnitine works by improving the uptake of fatty acids into the mitochondria (the energy organelle found in cells) for energy production. Studies in people and in animals (but not dogs) have shown an increase in weight loss and a reduction in lean tissue loss when L-carnitine is part of a low-calorie diet.

An effective dose is 50 mg to 300 mg of L-carnitine per kilogram (2.2 pounds) of food on a dry-matter basis. Talk to your veterinarian about how to supplement with L-carnitine.

Omega-3 Fatty Acids

Omega-3 fatty acids are one of the major supplements discussed in Chapter 1 and a supplement you may have read about in other chapters as well because it can provide many important benefits for your dog. Studies also suggest it can help with weight loss. Although most of the studies showing a weight loss advantage with omega-3s have been done in humans, at least one study was done in beagles. That study showed that dogs on a calorie-restricted diet lost more weight when their diet included omega-3 fatty acids. Research with rats have shown significant weight loss as well.

Fish oils—i.e., EPA (eicosapentaenoic acid) and DHA (docosahexaenoic acid)—are the most efficient and calorie-friendly way to provide omega-3 fatty acids to your dog's menu to help with weight loss. To achieve the level of omega-3 fatty acids needed to help with weight loss, you would need to give your dog much more of other oils that contain omega-3s, such as flaxseed and walnut oil. Since each teaspoon of oil contains 40 calories and you are trying to limit the amount of fat your dog consumes, you want to make sure you make each teaspoon count!

Consult your veterinarian for the optimal amount of omega-3 fish oil supplement containing both EPA and DHA for your dog. And remember: Because you will be adding extra calories to your dog's diet, you will need to subtract calories to make up the difference. However, the omega-3s will help serve two purposes: assist with weight loss, and help keep your dog's skin and haircoat healthy, which can be a problem when dogs are on low-fat diets.

Other Home Remedies

Dogs can get some help and support in the weight-loss department from a number of natural remedies. These supplements can be used along with your dietary and exercise program for weight loss.

- **Chromium picolinate.** This mineral can be helpful for dogs who have diabetes because it promotes the activity of insulin, and its usefulness in fighting excess weight in dogs has been suggested. Once again, discuss chromium supplementation with your veterinarian.

- **Conjugated linoleic acid (CLA).** The dietary component CLA has been shown to be helpful in weight loss in mice and humans, but so far no studies have been done in dogs. In mice, CLA helped increase weight loss and reduced body fat accumulation regardless of whether the mice were fed a high-fat or low-fat diet. In a 2012 human study, CLA reduced body weight, body mass index, and subcutaneous fat in overweight participants. Discuss the use of CLA for your overweight dog with your veterinarian before starting supplementation.
- **Dandelion.** The garden weed dandelion (*Taraxacum officinale*) is a bitter herb that is used as a mild diuretic, to support liver function, and to help with weight loss. Dandelion reportedly increases bile flow in animals, which in turn can improve fat metabolism. This herbal remedy is also rich in vitamins A, C, E, and the B-complex members, and a good source of potassium and calcium. No specific doses have been established for dogs, so you need to follow the recommendations of your veterinarian or use the "Herbal Doses for Dogs" guidelines on page 74. For example, a suggested dose of dandelion tincture (the easiest way to administer this herb) is 5 to 10 drops for each 10 pounds of your dog's weight, two to three times daily.
- **Kelp.** This supplement from the sea is often used to help with an underactive thyroid and may help restore your dog's metabolism. If your dog has hypothyroidism, ask your veterinarian about a seaweed supplement. Seaweed (*Fucus vesiculosus*) is a rich source of vitamins A, B, C, and D, and the minerals iron, magnesium, potassium, and zinc.

- **L-arginine.** This is another amino acid that has demonstrated an ability to reduce body fat, although the studies have not been done with dogs, only rats, pigs, and humans. All the studies also showed an increase in muscle mass when subjects took L-arginine. If your dog is having difficulty losing weight and you have not had success with other supplements, L-arginine may be helpful, especially if your dog needs to lose only a few pounds. Consult your veterinarian about the best dose for your dog.

Chapter 14

Upper Respiratory Infections

If you're a parent, you know that when there is a group of children, if one has the sniffles, it's not long before the germs are passed around. The same thing can happen with dogs and upper respiratory tract infections.

Upper respiratory infections affect a dog's eyes, throat, nose, and windpipe (trachea). They differ from lower respiratory infections, which have an impact on the smaller airways in the lungs and cause pneumonia.

Dogs at greatest risk of contracting an upper respiratory infection are those who have not been vaccinated for *Bordetella bronchiseptica* and who are in an environment that has many other dogs, such as a kennel or shelter, or puppies that have come from a pet store or similar facility. Elderly dogs and dogs who are not up-to-date on their other vaccinations are also at risk, as are dogs who have a compromised or weakened immune system, such as those with cancer or another chronic disease, or who eat a poor nutritional diet.

DOES MY DOG HAVE AN UPPER RESPIRATORY INFECTION?

The symptoms of an upper respiratory infection in dogs are strikingly similar to those of the common cold in people: sneezing, runny nose, coughing, and red, watery eyes. Your dog may also be less energetic, have a poor appetite, and have a fever. An infection that is caused by a virus usually is associated with a watery discharge from the nose and eyes, while those with a bacterial cause are typically associated with a thick, snotty discharge.

If the infection has moved into the lower respiratory tract, the common symptoms are coughing, wheezing, and trouble breathing. Fever, lack of appetite, and reduced activity are more common in dogs who have a lower respiratory infection than an infection that affects the upper respiratory tract. Without treatment, an upper respiratory infection can develop into a more serious infection or pneumonia. In short, upper respiratory infections are a widespread problem, but also one that can be treated effectively.

CAUSES OF UPPER RESPIRATORY INFECTIONS

The most common cause of upper respiratory infections in dogs are the bacteria *Bordetella bronchiseptica,* which cause a condition known as tracheobronchitis, or "kennel cough," with the characteristic hacking, almost gagging type of cough. Viruses also are culprits in upper respiratory infections, including the canine distemper virus (canine parainfluenza 3), canine herpes, and canine influenza. Viral infections can develop into a serious upper respiratory disease.

In cases of upper respiratory infections, the bacteria that normally reside in a dog's throat and mouth can become irritated by factors such as smoke, airborne allergens, dry air, or a viral infection. These irritants damage the tissues in the throat and mouth, which allows the bacteria to grow and multiply, especially in a dog with a compromised immune system.

Upper respiratory infections tend to be highly infectious, especially those caused by *Bordetella* and canine influenza. Therefore, if you have more than one dog in the house or your infected dog has opportunities to spend time with other dogs, she can easily spread the infection. However, people cannot catch upper respiratory infections from their dogs, nor can dogs catch upper respiratory infections from people. Vaccines are available for canine *Bordetella* and canine distemper, but none have yet been developed for canine influenza.

A tiny parasite appropriately called the nasal mite (*Pneumonyssoides caninum*) may also cause an upper respiratory infection. These mites are spread through direct dog-to-dog contact and can cause your dog to sneeze, cough, develop a chronic runny nose, and perhaps even experience nosebleeds. The presence of these mites increases the possibility of a bacterial or viral infection taking hold and causing an upper respiratory infection.

Infrequently, parasites called lung flukes can cause an upper respiratory infection. Lung flukes (*Paragonimus kellicotti*) live in cysts in the lungs of dogs, cats, and other mammals. To become infected, a dog must eat raw, infected crab or crayfish, or ingest part of an infected crayfish, which could happen if your dog drinks water from a lake or stream. Other causes of upper respiratory infection in dogs include sinusitis, rhinitis, and heartworm infection.

DIAGNOSING UPPER RESPIRATORY INFECTIONS

If your dog begins demonstrating symptoms of an upper respiratory infection, it's best to have her checked by a veterinarian as soon as possible to make sure the condition does not escalate into a more serious infection. This is especially important if you have a puppy who has come from a crowded environment or whose vaccination history you do not know. Young puppies do not have a fully developed immune system, which makes them especially vulnerable to infection.

Veterinarians usually diagnose an upper respiratory infection based on information from pet parents about the dog's recent exposures (e.g., kennel, doggie day care, and vaccination history), symptoms and clinical signs from listening to a dog's airways and lungs with a stethoscope, and possibly chest X-rays if there is suspicion of lower respiratory problems. Other conditions that have symptoms like those of an upper respiratory infection include lung tumors, a collapsed trachea, and tumors of the larynx, trachea, and nose.

CONVENTIONAL TREATMENT

Veterinarians frequently prescribe an antibiotic (tetracycline is the usual prescription) if a bacterial infection is suspected. This antibiotic can permanently stain the teeth of puppies. Other medications your veterinarian may prescribe include a cough suppressant, decongestant, or expectorant to provide your dog with some relief from her symptoms. Some human pediatric cold medications may be suitable for your dog, but do not give your dog anything unless you first consult with your veterinarian. If your dog has kennel cough, you should keep her away from other dogs so she doesn't spread the infection. Most cases of kennel cough last for one to two weeks.

Dogs with an upper respiratory infection should avoid excessive physical activity and be provided a nutritious diet and lots of fresh water. If the infection become severe or if it develops into a lower respiratory tract infection, your dog may need hospitalization for intravenous fluids or other medical support.

HOME REMEDIES

The importance of a nutritious diet that supports and maintains your dog's immune system is one of the main things you can do to help prevent upper respiratory infections. If you haven't upgraded your dog's diet yet, it's not too late to do it now (see chapter 3, "What's for Dinner? Good Food for Your Dog"). However, you probably are looking for home remedies to deal with a current infection, so let's get to it.

Home remedies can be completely effective in relieving symptoms and even eliminating an upper respiratory infection. However, if your dog's symptoms do not significantly improve after using home remedies for two to three days or if his symptoms worsen, see your veterinarian. You will likely be able to continue with your home remedies for symptom relief, but your dog may require medical intervention as well to prevent development of a more serious infection.

Chicken Soup

Yes, chicken soup just for your dog! You can actually get two uses out of the chicken: Cook the chicken for your dog or yourself, then remove all the bones for the soup. (No, there is no chicken meat in this soup.) You will need 1 pound of chicken bones, but if you have more, adjust the recipe accordingly.

1 lb chicken bones (You can use turkey bones.)
2 tbs apple cider vinegar
$1/2$ cup fresh parsley
8 cloves of garlic, mashed
4 celery stalks, chopped
4 large carrots, sliced
1 teaspoon salt

Place the bones in the bottom of a stock pot and add water until the bones are just covered. Add the vinegar and let the bones and water sit for an hour. Cover and simmer for five hours. Put the parsley into a piece of cheesecloth and tie tightly. Place the garlic, celery, carrots, parsley, and salt into the pot and return to a simmer for one hour. Remove the pot from heat and place a colander over a large bowl or pot to collect the broth. Pour the contents of the pot into the colander. Discard the bones and place the vegetables and parsley (take out of the cheesecloth) into a blender or food processor and puree. Add the purée to the broth. This chicken soup can be stored in the refrigerator tightly sealed for four to five days or freeze it for up to six months.

This soup can be the base for several remedies. For example, add $1/2$ to 1 teaspoon of honey to $1/4$ cup of the soup (lukewarm) and feed to your dog several times a day. You can also use the soup to deliver other powdered or liquid supplements to your dog.

Honey

Although there is no research demonstrating that honey can help cough in dogs, several studies in children have shown it to be beneficial. Honey also has antibacterial, antiviral, and anti-inflammatory properties, which are a bonus. Give your dog $1/2$ to 1 teaspoon of honey (use a runny honey if possible) three to four times a day. Most dogs have no problem lapping up this treat! If your dog is reluctant to lick the sticky honey, add the honey to a few ounces of warm water and put in his water bowl. If this fails, you can use a medicine dropper to put the honey solution into his mouth or add it to the chicken soup recipe provided in this section.

Vaporizer

Run a vaporizer in the room where your dog sleeps or spends most of her time. In the medicine holder, place any of the following to help relieve cough and to loosen phlegm: crushed cloves of garlic, essential oils of eucalyptus, lavender, or tea tree oil. A vaporizer is especially helpful for puppies who have kennel cough.

Vitamin C

According to Cheryl Schwartz, DVM, author of *Four Paws, Five Directions: A Guide to Chinese Medicine for Cats and Dogs*, a recommended dose of vitamin C for dogs with upper respiratory infection is 125 mg to 500 mg twice daily for small dogs, 250 mg to 1,500 mg twice daily for medium dogs, and 500 mg to 1,500 twice daily for large dogs. Vitamin C is a potent antioxidant that can help support the respiratory tract and immune system. The forms of vitamin C that are most easily absorbed in the intestinal tract are the ascorbates; that is, calcium ascorbate and sodium ascorbate. These forms of vitamin C also are less likely to cause diarrhea, which can occur if your dog takes too much vitamin C in one dose.

More Home Remedies

- **Peppermint.** Make a strong tea by steeping peppermint leaves in boiled water for thirty minutes, then cool. Add several drops of the cooled tea to 4 ounces of cooled water in your dog's water bowl. After your dog has finished this water, repeat with another 4 ounces of water plus the tea. This will help ensure your dog gets the tea. You can also add $\frac{1}{2}$ to 1 teaspoon of honey to the tea.
- **Probiotics.** These beneficial bacteria are recommended if your dog has been given antibiotics, because they will enhance and support the immune system and help restore the good bacteria destroyed by the antibiotics. Probiotics are a very safe supplement to give to your dog, and typical doses are in the hundreds of millions of colony-forming units

(CFUs). Probiotic products are available for dogs, so follow the supplement dosing directions. If you use a probiotic product for humans, give your dog the full suggested dose if he weighs 40 pounds or more, and reduce it accordingly if he weighs less. (See "Home Remedies" on page 134 for more on probiotics.)
- **Yerba santa.** This herb has expectorant and decongestant properties and can be used to make a strong tea. Administer the same way as you would the peppermint tea.

Chapter 15

Urinary Tract Infections

Has your ten-year-old collie mix Maggie started having little "accidents" in the house? Does your eight-year-old boxer mix Reginald whimper when he urinates? These dogs are showing signs of a urinary tract infection, a common condition that reportedly affects about 14 percent of dogs at any one time.

A urinary tract infection, also known as cystitis, is an infection that affects any part of the urinary tract, which includes the kidneys, ureters (tubes that transport urine from the kidneys to the bladder), urinary bladder, and urethra (the tube that transports urine from the bladder to the outside of the body). Female dogs are affected significantly more than are males because they have a much shorter urethra, which is the route the infectious agent takes to reach and infect the bladder.

DOES MY DOG HAVE A URINARY TRACT INFECTION?

Maggie and Reginald displayed two of the main signs of a urinary tract infection: a dog who starts to wet in the house, and painful urination. It's important to note, however, that dogs who have a urinary tract infection often don't show clinical signs of the condition. If they do, however, you may notice one or more of the following symptoms:

- abnormally frequent urination
- large volumes of urine

- urine leakage (incontinence, which may be noticeable if your dog is in the house a lot)
- blood in the urine
- increased thirst
- straining when urinating
- cloudy urine
- urine with an unusual smell
- lethargy
- lack of appetite
- fever
- irritation and/or inflammation around the external genitalia
- vaginal discharge (females)
- licking of the vulva (females)

Although it can be a challenge to identify urinary tract infections in dogs, it's important to treat them, because even uncomplicated asymptomatic cases (discussed under "Types and Causes of Urinary Tract Infections" on page 200), left untreated, can progress into serious conditions, including kidney infection and septicemia, a life-threatening condition involving bacteria in the blood.

WHICH DOGS ARE AT RISK FOR URINARY TRACT INFECTIONS?

We've already mentioned that female dogs are more susceptible to developing urinary tract infections, but other dogs also are at increased risk. For example, if your dog has been diagnosed with bladder or kidney stones or has a congenital or acquired structural defect in the urinary tract (e.g., dogs who are born with a narrow urethra), she is at greater risk of getting urinary tract infections. Long-term use of corticosteroids or other medications that suppress the immune system raise the possibility of developing urinary tract infections, as does having diabetes, hyperadenocorticism

(Cushing's disease), or a number of other disorders (see below).

TYPES AND CAUSES OF URINARY TRACT INFECTIONS

Dogs typically get urinary tract infections when bacteria invade the urethra and make their way into the bladder. The bacteria most often involved are E. coli, staphylococcus, proteus, enterococcus, klebsiella, streptococcus, enterobacterium, chlamydia and pseudomonas. Despite this long list of possible culprits, only one bacterial species is usually involved when a dog gets ill. Infrequently, fungi (e.g., candida, *Cryptococcus neoformans*, *Rhodotorula*, *Trichosporon*), viruses, algae, or mycoplasma can cause a urinary tract infection.

After the culprits enter the urethra and the bladder, they may also expand their invasion to the ureters and kidneys, in which case there is great potential for a life-threatening systemic infection. That's why it's critical to nip a urinary tract infection in the bud before it spreads.

Urinary tract infections in dogs can be simple and uncomplicated or persistent and complicated. Let's start with the simple form.

Nearly all uncomplicated urinary tract infections in dogs are caused by bacteria and have no underlying structural or functional abnormalities that are behind the infection (e.g., a congenital deformity of the urinary tract). In most cases, just one type of bacteria is responsible for the infection, although mixed infections do occur. Rarely, viruses, fungi, chlamydia, or mycoplasma may cause an uncomplicated urinary tract infection.

The prognosis for dogs who have uncomplicated urinary tract infections caused by bacteria is excellent. Those who have a fungal cause, however, are difficult to treat.

Complicated or recurrent urinary tract infections are those that are caused by a structural defect or a disorder, such as a bladder tumor or polyps, prostatitis (an inflamed prostate gland), pyelonephritis (kidney infection), kidney failure, cancer, diabetes, long-term corticosteroid use, hyperadrenocorticism, and bladder stones. Because female dogs are much more likely to develop a urinary tract infection associated with bacteria (the uncomplicated infection), male dogs who have a urinary tract infection typically are diagnosed with a complicated form.

Complicated urinary tract infections are more difficult to diagnose and treat than uncomplicated cases because veterinarians must first identify and resolve the underlying problem. For example, for dogs who have diabetes, which is associated with recurrent urinary tract infections, tight control of blood and urine glucose levels is critical to prevent such urinary problems. Therefore the prognosis for dogs with complicated urinary tract infections varies and depends on how well the underlying cause is managed or resolved and accurately identifying the organism involved.

DIAGNOSING URINARY TRACT INFECTIONS

A key tool to help diagnose a urinary tract infection is a routine urinalysis. Your veterinarian likely won't ask Rufus to pee into a cup, however. A urine collection method called cystocentesis is often performed, and it involves inserting a sterile needle into the bladder and taking a urine sample using a syringe. The urine is then evaluated using chemical analysis, urine specific gravity, microscopic evaluation, and visual examination. All the information gathered, including urine pH (whether the urine is acidic or alkaline) and levels of protein, ketones, bilirubin, blood, nitrites, glucose, bacteria, yeast, and other substances and organisms, are clues veterinarians can use to determine the function of the kidneys and other organs and to help identify possible causes of the urinary tract infection.

The urine sample can also be used to do a urine culture, during which the sample is placed in growth media and monitored over a few days to look for bacterial, fungal, viral, or yeast growth to identify the organism that is causing the infection.

Don't be surprised if your veterinarian also wants to do a complete blood count and serum chemistry profile, both of which will help uncover underlying conditions such as cancer, kidney disease, or hyperadrenocorticism. Complicated cases of urinary tract infection may require abdominal X-rays to look for tumors, stones, an enlarged prostate gland, or unusual sediment in the bladder. Abdominal ultrasound may be ordered to evaluate the anatomy of the kidneys, urethra, and bladder.

CONVENTIONAL TREATMENT

Typically, dogs with a urinary tract infection are treated with antibiotics for two to three weeks based on the results of the urinalysis and blood tests. One or more antibiotics may be ordered. A urine culture is often done five to seven days after you complete the course of antibiotics to make sure the infection has been eliminated. If the infection does not resolve or if it returns after the antibiotic course is done, then a urine culture is usually done and a new antibiotic course may be chosen. The veterinarian will also treat any underlying cause of the urinary tract infection that has been identified.

HOME REMEDIES

Urinary tract infections generally are not life-threatening and in many cases can be handled effectively using home remedies (with advice from your veterinarian of course) unless the occurrence is severe. The following home remedies are suggested for cases of urinary tract infections that are considered to be mild to moderate.

Apple Cider Vinegar

Apple cider vinegar works well in people who have urinary tract infections, but the positive reports in dogs are purely anecdotal. However, vinegar is proven to neutralize bacteria in urine and is safe. Try adding ½ teaspoon of apple cider vinegar to your dog's food once a day or putting it into her water bowl for three to four days in row.

Citrus Juice

When you have your morning orange juice, perhaps your dog can join you. Citrus juices such as orange juice, grapefruit juice, and lemon juice can enhance the acidity of your dog's urine, which in turn can reduce the bacteria level. Try 4 to 8 ounces per day, depending on the size of your dog. You can add it to her water bowl.

Vitamin C

Dogs are capable of making their own vitamin C, but extra doses of this water-soluble antioxidant may help in fighting urinary tract infections. Daily doses of vitamin C are recommended by Cheryl Schwartz, DVM, author of *Four Paws, Five Directions: A Guide to Chinese Medicine for Cats and Dogs*. The suggested dose is 125 mg twice a day for small dogs, 250 mg twice daily for medium dogs, and 500 mg twice a day for large dogs. The forms of vitamin C best absorbed by the intestinal tract are calcium ascorbate and sodium ascorbate; they are also are less likely to cause diarrhea, which can occur if your dog takes too much vitamin C at one time.

Water

As in people who have urinary tract infections, it is important to drink lots of water to flush out the bacteria. Ways to encourage your dog to drink more water may be to add citrus juices to her water or to float ice cubes in the water to keep it cool.

Chapter 16

Vomiting and Gastritis

"Hey, Mom, the dog threw up!" "Oh, no, the dog puked on the carpet!" "I think the dog barfed!" Plenty of pet parents have heard these words or uttered similar ones on their own. My personal "favorite" is waking up in the middle of the night and stepping into you-know-what in bare feet. If only your dog knew to head for the toilet bowl when he didn't feel well.

Vomiting is one of the most common symptoms dogs experience, and it is also one of the main symptoms of gastritis, one of the most common digestive disorders that affects dogs. Although dogs often experience vomiting that has nothing to do with gastritis, both of these health issues often occur in dogs and the association between the two is strong, so they warrant discussion in the same chapter.

What both vomiting and gastritis naturally have in common is that they both involve the stomach, so let's take a quick look at how the canine stomach works.

CANINE STOMACH

Your dog's stomach, like yours, is designed to store food and fluids while they go through a digestive process and then are sent on their way into the small intestine. Food enters your dog's stomach through a valvelike structure called the cardiac sphincter. Once in the stomach, the food is ground by structures called gastric folds while the inner stomach lining secretes acids and enzymes that break down the food so the nutrients can be more easily absorbed once they reach the small intestine.

This completes the stomach's role in digestion, so the partially digested food leaves the stomach through the pyloric sphincter and enters the first part of the small intestine, called the duodenum. Most of the food your dog eats leaves his stomach within twelve hours after entering.

Sometimes, however, something goes wrong, and the food makes a U-turn and leaves via the same route it entered the stomach.

VOMITING

"Vomiting," "barfing," "puking," "throwing up"—all are terms commonly used to describe the forceful expulsion of the stomach's contents through the mouth. There's a difference between vomiting and regurgitation, however. When a dog vomits, the stomach muscles undergo several strong contractions that can involve the entire body. These contractions force the food out of the stomach and through the esophagus and mouth. Regurgitated food has never reached the stomach; therefore your dog will not experience the muscle contractions if she regurgitates her food.

IS THE VOMITING SERIOUS?

A common question is: "If my dog is vomiting, when is it serious enough to call my veterinarian?" Generally, if your dog vomits once or even twice and you've watched him closely and he is alert and energetic, then you probably do not need to call your veterinarian. He likely ate some grass or perhaps finished his dinner too quickly.

However, if your dog vomits and you can answer "Yes" to one or more of the following questions, then you should call your veterinarian. When you make the call, it would help your veterinarian if you could also tell her when the vomiting started, how many times your dog has vomited, and what the vomit looks like (color, consistency, any blood).

- ✓ Do you think your dog has eaten something poisonous or dangerous?
- ✓ Is there blood in the vomit?
- ✓ Does your dog's stomach look bloated?
- ✓ Are his gums pale or yellow?
- ✓ Does your dog have diarrhea?
- ✓ Is your dog a puppy who has not had all his vaccinations?
- ✓ Is your dog acting like he is in pain?
- ✓ Does your dog have dry heaves (acting like he is going to vomit but cannot)?

CAUSES AND DIAGNOSIS OF VOMITING

As I mentioned earlier, vomiting is one of the main symptoms of gastritis, but it can also be a symptom or result of many other conditions and situations (see "Causes of Vomiting" page 208). Some of the causes result in minor episodes of vomiting and require minor action on your part, while others are more serious and demand immediate medical attention. Therefore it's important to identify the cause of the vomiting so the appropriate treatment can be offered.

CAUSES OF VOMITING

- gastritis
- ulcers
- parasites
- change in diet
- food intolerance
- eating garbage or other inappropriate items such as dirt or paper
- poison (e.g., antifreeze, pesticides, household chemicals)
- gastrointestinal condition such as inflammatory bowel disease or colitis
- bacterial or viral infection
- diabetes
- organ disease: liver disease, kidney disease, peritonitis, pancreatitis, Addison's disease
- gastroesophageal reflux
- motion sickness (See "Motion Sickness in Dogs" on facing page.)
- medications

If you have identified the cause of the vomiting (for example, you caught Duchess finishing off last night's dinner in the trash can), then the detective work is done. However, if more sleuthing is required, your veterinarian can conduct an examination and ask questions, such as:

- When did the vomiting start?
- Did your dog vomit or regurgitate?
- What does the vomit look like? Does it contain bile, blood, pieces of food, bone, or any identifiable materials?

- Does your dog smack or lick her lips, drool, gulp, or swallow? (These signs indicate that your dog is nauseous.)
- How often does your dog vomit?
- Is the vomiting violent (i.e., projectile vomiting)?
- Does your dog have any signs of pain, weakness, diarrhea, weight loss, fever, changes in urination, loss of appetite?

Your veterinarian will conduct a physical examination and also ask about your dog's medical history, including vaccinations, any medications, diet, access to poisons or garbage, contact with other dogs, and parasite history. In some cases, tests may be done on a stool sample to check for worms, bacterial infection, parvovirus, or other infections. A complete blood count and chemistry panel may be recommended as well. If your veterinarian suspects an anatomical problem or tumor, imaging tests such as ultrasound or X-rays may be ordered.

MOTION SICKNESS IN DOGS

Some dogs love to ride in a car or stand on the deck of a fishing boat, but others experience bouts of motion sickness from these adventures. Motion sickness is more common in puppies and young dogs because the ear structures involved with balance are not yet fully developed. Many dogs outgrow motion sickness, although puppies who vomited when riding in a car may be conditioned to associate the car with vomiting and resist trips as they get older. Possible causes of motion sickness in mature dogs include stress, associating the car with a previous bad experience, and fear of confined spaces.

(continued)

Signs of motion sickness include yawning, whining, excessive drooling, vomiting, and restlessness. Antinausea medications, antihistamines, phenothiazine, and similar drugs may be given to dogs who don't respond to nondrug approaches, which should be tried first. They include:

- ✓ **Water.** Make sure your dog is well hydrated before going in the car, but withhold food for about three hours before the ride.
- ✓ **Ginger.** Give your dog a small piece of ginger candy or a ginger supplement (500-mg capsule) about thirty minutes before going out in the car.
- ✓ **Peppermint.** Prepare peppermint tea and allow it to cool. Give some cooled peppermint tea to your dog about thirty minutes before you take a ride and bring extra tea with you in case your dog gets sick in the car.
- ✓ **Valerian.** Valerian is a calming herb, so if your dog is anxious or stressed, add a few drops of tincture of valerian to her water bowl before your trip.

GASTRITIS

Gastritis is inflammation ("-itis") of the stomach ("gastric") lining. One of the main symptoms of gastritis is vomiting, and the characteristics of the vomiting are important to note for your veterinarian, so let's look more closely at those traits as well as other symptoms of gastritis:

- **vomiting.** It may be sudden and extreme in acute gastritis or persistent and severe in chronic cases.

The vomit may be frothy and yellowish in color (indicating the presence of bile), have specks of red blood, and/or contain digested blood, which looks like coffee grounds.

- **abdominal pain.** The pain can range from mild to severe and be debilitating. Your dog may stand with his head hanging down as if he were bowing.
- **loss of appetite**
- **diarrhea**
- **weakness and lethargy**
- **fever** (temperature higher than 101.5 degrees)
- **dehydration**
- **blood in the stool** (not common)
- **yellowish or pale gums** (usually associated with ingesting toxins)
- **excessive drooling** (usually associated with ingesting toxins)
- **dull haircoat**

IS MY DOG AT RISK FOR GASTRITIS?

Gastritis can develop in dogs of any breed, age, or gender. If your dog has access to and enjoys rummaging in garbage or is fond of ingesting animal feces, plant matter (including grass), and/or foreign objects such as string, plastic, or other indigestible material, these habits place him or her at increased risk of causing irritation and inflammation of the gastrointestinal tract. A type of gastritis called hypertrophic pyloric gastropathy is seen in small, flat-faced breeds, such as Boston terriers, bulldogs, and pugs, as well as basenjis, Lhasa apsos, miniature poodles, and shih tzus. This condition occurs in middle-aged dogs and causes the dogs to vomit a few hours after they eat. Chronic hypertrophic pyloric gastropathy is caused by a narrowing of the pyloric canal, the area of the stomach that connects with the first part of the small intestine.

TYPES AND CAUSES OF GASTRITIS

Gastritis can occur in two forms: acute or chronic. The good news about both types of gastritis is that although they will make your dog uncomfortable, most cases are not serious and are treatable, even though for many dogs the cause of their gastrointestinal discomfort is never identified.

That said, regardless of the cause, most dogs who develop gastritis respond well to treatment and can be managed well at home with guidance from their veterinarian as needed. (See "Conventional Treatment" on page 214 and "Home Remedies" on page 215.)

Now let's look at the two types of gastritis and their causes.

Acute Gastritis

Acute gastritis comes on suddenly and nearly always involves persistent vomiting and severe abdominal pain. Dogs typically get acute gastritis for the following reasons:

- ingesting poisonous substances, such as antifreeze, rat poison, fertilizers, or household chemicals
- ingesting irritating medications (Some dogs react to nonsteroidal anti-inflammatory drugs, antibiotics, aspirin, and antibiotics.)
- serious organ disease, such as kidney failure, liver failure, pancreatitis (inflamed pancreas) or Addison's disease (hypoadrenocorticism, or failure of the adrenal glands)
- internal parasites
- overeating or binge eating (e.g., dogs who "wolf down" their food)
- eating inappropriate things (e.g., garbage, moldy

food, toxic household plants, socks, feces of other dogs or animals)
- bacterial or viral infections

Chronic Gastritis

Most causes of acute gastritis can also lead to chronic gastritis, and one reason is timing. Chronic gastritis is caused by persistent, long-term irritation of the bacterial environment and mucosal lining of the digestive tract. For example, if your dog has a habit of eating paper or string, these items can continuously irritate her digestive tract, increasingly causing inflammation of the stomach lining and resulting in chronic gastritis. A bacterial infection that is not treated and resolved promptly can become a prolonged problem, again resulting in chronic gastritis.

Other common causes of chronic gastritis include food allergies, chemical irritants, cancer, liver disease, and kidney disease. Puppies can get chronic gastritis if they have not been vaccinated for parvovirus. Intestinal parasites and stomach polyps are other possible causes, while stress can be a contributing factor.

DIAGNOSING GASTRITIS

The initial evaluation will include a thorough physical examination by your veterinarian. You can help with the diagnosis if you provide as much information as possible about your dog's vomiting and other symptoms, as well as his diet, access to garbage and other items he may have eaten, and use of medications.

Veterinarians typically rule out as many possible causes of a dog's symptoms as possible to try and identify the cause of gastritis, but often the underlying cause is never identified.

Most cases of gastritis are associated with "dietary indiscretion," which means the dog ate something he should have avoided. In such cases, veterinarians recommend withholding food for a day or two and offering the dog water only (see "Conventional Treatment" below).

Dogs who do not respond to this initial diagnosis can undergo blood and urine tests and possibly imaging tests of the abdomen. Blood tests can be especially helpful in ruling out a wide range of illnesses, such as diabetes, liver disease, kidney disease, parvovirus, and endocrine disorders. X-rays and ultrasound can identify the presence of any blockages or defects in the gastrointestinal tract. Infrequently, tissue biopsies are taken of the stomach lining to look for infectious microorganisms.

CONVENTIONAL TREATMENT

Treating your dog for a mild case of vomiting or gastritis is much like treating a child with the same condition: Withhold food for about twenty-four hours to allow her stomach to settle down, make sure she has enough water given often but in small amounts, and then give her a bland diet for several days (for vomiting) or two to three weeks (for gastritis) until her gastrointestinal tract has had a chance to heal. (See "Home Remedies" on facing page for recipe ideas.) For some dogs, vomiting may be a sign of a food intolerance, so a permanent change in diet may be necessary after some experimentation with an elimination diet (see chapter 5, "Atopic Dermatitis").

Avoid the impulse to reach into your medicine cabinet and treat your dog with Pepto-Bismol without first consulting with your veterinarian, even though this medication is one of the few that is recommended for both dogs and people. Although best known as an antidiarrheal drug, the pink thick liquid can also soothe your dog's irritated stomach caused by vomiting and something your dog ate. The typical dose is

0.5 to 1 ml of Pepto-Bismol per pound of body weight given every six to eight hours.

Use a plastic syringe to squirt the medicine into the back of your dog's mouth to avoid having your dog shake the pink liquid out of her mouth. Pepto-Bismol is also available as tablets. A possible side effect is black-colored stools, while some dogs cannot tolerate silicates and so will not benefit from the medication.

Another medication for vomiting and diarrhea, called loperamide (Immodium), is safe for dogs. A typical dose is 1 teaspoon every four to six hours for every 20 pounds of body weight.

For dogs with more serious symptoms, such as persistent vomiting, diarrhea, fever, and dehydration, intravenous fluids may be necessary to replace lost fluids and electrolytes (sodium, potassium, chloride, bicarbonate). Prescription medication to reduce vomiting, such as aminopentamide (Centrine), may be recommended to reduce acidity in the stomach and relieve spasms in the gastrointestinal tract. Your veterinarian may prescribe antibiotics if vomiting or gastritis is caused by a bacterial infection. Several studies have shown the prescription drugs famotidine and omeprazole to be helpful in exercise-induced gastritis, particularly in sled dogs. Before any medications are given, however, it's important to have an accurate diagnosis.

If your dog's gastritis is caused by an indigestible object that is stuck in your dog's stomach or upper small intestine, then surgery may be necessary.

HOME REMEDIES

Home remedies for dogs who experience vomiting and/or gastritis include a diet and supplements that will gently restore the function of their gastrointestinal tract. Here are a few suggestions:

Probiotics

Supplements that provide beneficial bacteria, or probiotics, can help relieve your dog's upset stomach and vomiting caused by gastritis, dietary changes, a bacterial or viral infection, exposure to toxins or certain medications, or eating things she shouldn't have. Probiotics work by restoring a healthy balance of bacteria in the gastrointestinal tract, which can be thrown out of balance when dogs experience vomiting and gastritis. (See "Probiotics" on page 136.) Probiotic supplements that provide a variety of different species and strains are recommended. The main species and strains of beneficial bacteria belong to five main genera: bacillus, bifidobacterium, enterococcus, lactobacillus, and streptococcus.

In addition to the many pet parents and veterinarians who have witnessed how well their dogs respond to probiotics, there is also some limited research on the subject. One study appeared in the January 2010 issue of the *Journal of Small Animal Practice*. Dogs who were experiencing gastroenteritis (acute diarrhea or acute diarrhea and vomiting) were treated with placebo or probiotics (*Lactobacillus acidophilus*, *L. farciminis*, *Pediococcus acidilactici*, *Bacillus subtilis*, *B. licheniformis*). The probiotics reduced the amount of time the dogs experienced diarrhea (from an average of 2.2 days to 1.3 days), although the treatment and placebo groups were similar regarding the time from start of treatment to the last vomiting episode.

Probiotic supplements specially formulated for dogs are available in powder, liquid, and pills. Look for products that contain five or more species and strains, because the more opportunities you provide your dog's gastrointestinal system to heal, the better. Some probiotic supplements need to be refrigerated, so be sure to check the storage directions.

How much probiotics should you give your dog? Exact doses have not been determined, but since probiotics are very safe, you don't need to worry about overdosing your dog. Follow the recommendations from your veterinarian or the instructions on the supplement. If you use a probiotic product for humans, give the full recommended dose to your dog if she weighs 40 pounds or more, and reduce the dose if she weighs less.

Bland Diet

A standard treatment for dogs who are suffering with vomiting or gastritis is a bland diet. After you have allowed your dog's digestive tract to "calm down" for twenty-four to forty-eight hours by withholding food, you need to slowly reintroduce foods that will hopefully not cause distress. If your dog experienced acute vomiting but not gastritis, you can generally feed her a bland diet for several days and then gradually reintroduce her regular diet. Dogs with gastritis may need to follow a bland diet for two weeks or longer. Consult with your veterinarian.

Here are a few suggestions for a bland diet. Feed your dog her normal daily allotment of food, but divide it into smaller portions to allow her digestive system to return to normal. Provide your dog with a tablespoon of plain nonfat yogurt after each meal.

Nonmeat Protein Recipe

8 ounces of cooked brown rice or barley
8 ounces of farmer cheese
1 egg, boiled and mashed
1 teaspoon vegetable oil
1 gram calcium carbonate
multivitamin/mineral supplement

Combine all ingredients and feed in appropriate portions, depending on the size of your dog.

Chicken Recipe for Gastritis

8 ounces cooked chicken, no skin or fat
8 ounces cooked barley or quinoa
$1/2$ cup cooked pumpkin
1 gram calcium carbonate
multivitamin/mineral supplement

Combine all ingredients and feed in appropriate portions, depending on the size of your dog.

Other Home Remedies

- **Chamomile.** Two drops of chamomile tincture per pound of your dog's body weight in his water three times a day may help with an upset stomach.
- **Ginger.** This herb is a popular natural treatment for nausea and vomiting in people, and it has been reported to work in dogs as well. A 2012 study in the *Journal of Alternative and Complementary Medicine* reported that ginger was effective in relieving vomiting in dogs subjected to cancer chemotherapy. Anecdotal reports say ginger may help with motion sickness. For relief of vomiting and gastritis, you might give your dog 1 drop of ginger tincture per pound of body weight twice daily in her water after consulting your veterinarian.

Chapter 17

Worms (Intestinal Parasites)

One of the least pleasant and often misunderstood problems that affect dogs is worms. The least pleasant designation is self-explanatory: There's a significant "yuck" factor when you think about the creatures wiggling around in your dog, seeing the pieces of worms in doggie poop, and collecting said poop for your vet to examine.

However, yucky or not, intestinal parasites can be a serious health problem for your dog, so it's best to understand them and what you can do about these pests. Among the misconceptions are the belief that only puppies can get worms and that dogs can get worms from drinking milk. A serious misconception is that you'll know when your dog has worms because you will see them.

This is not always true. In fact, of the four main types of intestinal worms that can affect your dog, it is possible for you to see only two of them without the aid of a microscope, but it is also possible the stool samples you look at won't contain any worms even if your dog has worms.

So feel free to check your dog's stool, especially if you have a puppy, but it's still recommended that your veterinarian perform a fecal exam for your dog once a year. Naturally, you should always be aware of any symptoms of worms your dog may display, which may trigger a trip to the vet before that once-a-year checkup.

DOES MY DOG HAVE WORMS?

If your dog has worms, he or she may experience one or more of the following symptoms: diarrhea (may be bloody), weight loss, gas, gastrointestinal pain, dry hair, vomiting (there may be worms in the vomit), and failure to thrive (especially in puppies). However, your dog could have worms and experience no symptoms, or worm eggs and larvae may remain inactive in your dog's body until the dog experiences stress. For example, the latter stages of pregnancy can activate roundworms and hookworms so they infect the soon-to-arrive puppies.

Each type of intestinal parasite can cause different symptoms. Puppies and young dogs who are severely infested with roundworms, for example, typically have a potbelly and a poor coat. Dogs who are infested with hookworms are usually fatigued and have anemia. When tapeworms take hold, dogs may drag their rear ends along the ground, while dogs who are infested with whipworms may have no signs or symptoms other than black diarrhea.

TYPES OF WORMS

Here's the skinny on the intestinal worms most likely to affect dogs.

Roundworms

Roundworms (*Toxocara canis*, *T. leonina*) are the most common worm parasites in dogs and almost a fact of life for puppies, who typically get the microscopic roundworm larvae directly from their mothers, either through the uterus or from her milk. In addition to prenatal infection with roundworms and infection via mother's milk, a dog can become infected with ascarids by ingesting eggs in the soil or eating an infested mouse or other rodent.

Roundworms invade the intestinal tract and set up camp, growing up to seven inches long and shedding eggs in the intestinal tract. Those eggs can be passed out of the dog via feces, but others hatch into microscopic larvae that migrate to the lungs, where they are coughed up, swallowed, and make their way to the small intestine.

Puppies who have roundworms often have a potbelly and experience poor growth. If the worms are not treated in time, they can block the intestinal tract and cause death. Dogs older than six months develop an acquired resistance to roundworms, but that doesn't mean the worms are gone. In fact, the larvae become encased in a shell and take hold in various tissues throughout the body. The shell protects the larvae from the dog's antibodies and from most deworming medication.

However, if you have a female dog and you plan to allow her to get pregnant, you should know that pregnancy activates the encysted larvae, allowing them to move to the placenta and mammary glands, where they position themselves to infect the puppies. Therefore, it is important to deworm a female before pregnancy, which will reduce (but not eliminate) the larvae.

Whipworms

Whipworms (*Trichuris vulpis, T. campanula*) are threadlike creatures that grow up to three inches in length and are thicker at one end, which makes them look like a whip. They are common in dogs throughout the United States, and once they infect a dog, they live in the large intestine and cecum (junction of the small and large intestines). Dogs can become infected with whipworms by ingesting food or water that has been contaminated with whipworm eggs.

Once a dog swallows whipworm eggs, they hatch and

develop into adults in about three months. The adults burrow into the walls of the cecum and large intestine and feed on blood, but they are also busy laying eggs. Whipworm eggs leave the dog's body in feces, and these eggs must remain in the soil for about thirty days to mature and be capable of infecting other dogs. That's why it's important to pick up after your dog, both in your yard and in public areas.

Whipworms can be a challenge to diagnose because they are not often seen in the feces and the adult worms do not shed a lot of eggs. Therefore, sometimes a veterinarian must examine several stool samples before whipworms can be identified.

If your pooch has whipworms, he or she may experience acute, chronic, or off-and-on diarrhea that is bloody and covered with mucus. Some dogs experience bleeding of the intestinal tract, anemia, and weight loss.

Hookworms

The name of these worms gives away how they attach themselves to the intestinal wall and suck blood from dogs. Hookworms (*Ancylostoma caninum*) are typically less than 1 inch long, but they can suck enough blood and fluids from puppies to result in severe blood loss and malnutrition. Active worms leave bite sites, and those sites continue to bleed once the worms have moved on.

Puppies can become infected with hookworms from the uterus of their mother, from eating soil contaminated with the larvae, from their mother's milk, or if the worms burrow through the pads of the feet. Puppies and older dogs with hookworms look unhealthy and have a poor appetite, and the linings of their lips, ears, and nostrils are pale. If the hookworms make their way into the lungs, the dog will develop a cough and also experience diarrhea, tarry stools, and constipation. A severe infection can cause death in puppies as well as older dogs if not treated immediately.

Tapeworms

Tapeworms (*Dipylidium caninum*) are parasites that have a small head with many tiny egg-filled segments attached, resulting in a worm that can grow from several inches up to a foot or longer within the intestinal tract. Dogs can get tapeworms if they ingest fleas or they interact with wildlife that are infested with tapeworms or fleas. Therefore, measures to help prevent tapeworm infestations are to keep your dog away from dead or injured wildlife, avoid feeding raw meat (which may contain tapeworm eggs), and always treat for fleas (see chapter 11, "Fleas and Ticks").

Young dogs with tapeworm infestations may have diarrhea and vomiting. One telltale sign your dog may have tapeworms is if he scoots around with his rear end on the ground. The most common way to diagnose tapeworm is to find the worm segments. When the segments dry, they look like grains of rice, which can be seen in a dog's stool or clinging to the fur around the dog's rear end. However, since tapeworm eggs are eliminated in segments, a single fecal examination can miss an infestation.

CONVENTIONAL TREATMENT

As always, prevention is the best treatment. Therefore, always treat your dog for fleas; do not allow your dog to capture, play with, or eat wildlife; clean up after your dog (time to invest in that pooper scooper); and don't allow your dog to eat feces (including her own). That said, dogs still do get worms, and so the conventional way to ensure you have eliminated worms in your dog is to treat her with medication.

Numerous brands of worm medications are available both over-the-counter (OTC) and by prescription from your veterinarian, and each one has its own specific dosing instructions.

For this reason, and because every dog has different needs and health issues, get a clear diagnosis before you treat your dog and always consult your veterinarian before using any type of dewormer or worm medicine.

Here are some examples of worm medications. Some products are effective against more than one type of worm. Note the side effects.

- **Drontal Plus.** This prescription-only medication can treat tapeworms, hookworms, and whipworms. Dosage is based on your dog's weight, and the tablets are scored. Active ingredients are praziquantel, pyrantel pamoate, and febantel, and possible side effects include vomiting, loss of appetite, and diarrhea.
- **D-Worm Dog Wormer.** This OTC product is for roundworms and hookworms and available as a chewable tablet. Only one dose is required. The active ingredient is pyrantel pamoate. No side effects were reported in clinical trials.
- **HomeoPet Wrm Clear.** This is an all-natural liquid homeopathic worm medicine that reportedly helps eliminate hookworms, roundworms, and tapeworms. It can be added to your dog's water or placed directly into her mouth for seven days. No side effects have been reported.
- **Nemex-2.** This is a liquid dewormer available by prescription for large roundworms and hookworms. Puppies typically need a series of treatments, depending on their age at diagnosis. The active ingredient is pyrantel pamoate. Side effects are not common, but vomiting may occur.
- **Panacur C.** This dewormer can eliminate all four main types of worms. The drug is administered for three consecutive days and the dose is based on your dog's weight. The active ingredient is fenbendazole,

and possible side effects include loose stools, nausea, and vomiting.

- **Safe-Guard.** This OTC product is for dogs older than six weeks of age and can eliminate all four major types of worms. The medication should be given for three days in your dog's food, and the dose is determined by your dog's weight. Fenbendazole is the active ingredient, and possible side effects include loose stools, nausea, and vomiting.

- **Sentinel.** This prescription-only worm medication protects against adult roundworms, adult hookworms, whipworms, and heartworms (not discussed in this chapter), while also preventing the development of flea eggs. This flea protection is important because if your dog ingests fleas that are infected with tapeworms, your dog will get tapeworms. Sentinel is available as flavored tablets and is given once a month in the dog's food. The active ingredients are lufenuron and milbemycin oxime, and possible side effects include depression, diarrhea, drowsiness, hives, itching, loss of appetite, seizures, or vomiting.

- **Wormout.** This is an OTC product for both dogs and cats that can eliminate hookworms, whipworms, tapeworms, and roundworms. Treatment involves giving your dog six tablets to ensure the eggs, larvae, and worms are eliminated. Wormout can be given to dogs older than two weeks old, and the dose is determined by your dog's weight. The manufacturer (Vetafarm) recommends treating dogs every three months with the product. Active ingredients: oxibendazole and praziquantel.

- **WormX Plus.** This is an OTC chewable tablet that comes in two different sizes for easy dosing. WormX Plus eliminates hookworms, whipworms, and tapeworms and can be used on dogs and puppies age twelve weeks and older and weighing six pounds or more. The tablets contain pyrantel pamoate and praziquantel, which may cause diarrhea, loss of appetite, and vomiting.

HOME REMEDIES

A combination of a natural food diet (see chapters 2, "Is Dog Food Fit for Your Dog?" and 3, "What's for Dinner? Good Food for Your Dog"), natural supplements, and preventive measures can be an effective home remedy approach for preventing and eliminating worms, especially if your dog has a mild case of these intestinal pests. Consider the following home remedies for the prevention and/or elimination of intestinal worms.

Cloves and Fennel

The combination of cloves and fennel—and you can add garlic as well—has long been used to treat intestinal worm infestations in puppies. Cloves are the unopened flower buds of the evergreen clove tree, which are then dried. An active ingredient in cloves, called eugenol, has antibacterial properties and has been used to help prevent toxicity from environmental pollutants. Fennel (*Foeniculum vulgare*) is a perennial herb that looks like dill. The herbal remedies made from dried fennel seeds and leaves have long been used to help prevent and treat intestinal worms.

A mixture of one minced clove of garlic along with one teaspoon of crushed fennel and a pinch of ground cloves, added to your puppy's food, can help eliminate worms through your dog's feces.

Diatomaceous Earth

Diatomaceous earth is a nontoxic substance made from the ground-up fossils of freshwater organisms and marine life. Although diatomaceous earth appears to be a fine powder, a microscopic view will reveal that the powder is actually composed of sharp-edged particles that can be deadly to intestinal worms and their larvae because the sharp edges break through their protective coating so they dehydrate and die. However, the microscopic sharp edges do not harm pets or people.

If you use diatomaceous earth to treat your dog for worms, make sure you buy food-grade diatomaceous earth. **WARNING: The type of diatomaceous earth used for gardening and pool filters can harm your dog.** To eliminate hookworms, roundworms, or whipworms, just add about 1 teaspoon per 25 pounds of body weight to your dog's food per day and she won't even know it's in there, because diatomaceous earth is odorless and tasteless. For the best effect, give diatomaceous earth to your dog every day for at least thirty days so you can make sure to catch the worms throughout their life cycles. You may also want to keep diatomaceous earth around to deal with fleas and mites (see chapter 11, "Fleas and Ticks").

Garlic

Along with being a natural antibiotic and an immune system booster, garlic also helps get rid of worms. Garlic contains sulfur compounds and other nutrients that have medicinal value, including allicin and alliin. Dr. Cathy Alinovi recommends a dose of 1 clove of garlic (crushed or minced) added to your dog's food throughout the day in six portions. Large dogs (more than 35 pounds) can be given 2 to 3 cloves daily. If your dog doesn't like the taste of garlic (and some dogs do not), be sure to add each portion to something your dog really enjoys.

No specific scientific studies of the effect of garlic on worms in dogs have been conducted, but garlic has proven effective in eliminating hookworms and roundworms in people and in eliminating intestinal parasites in mice.

Pumpkin Seeds

Pumpkin seeds (*Cucurbita pepo*) are a traditional remedy for roundworms and tapeworms in dogs. Fresh, raw pumpkin seeds (no husks) can be ground and added to your dog's food. A suggested dose is ¼ to 1 teaspoon per 10 to 20 pounds of body weight at each meal for two to three weeks.

What makes pumpkin seeds a worm fighter? They contain an amino acid called cucurbitin, which has antiworm properties: it can paralyze and eliminate worms from the digestive tract in both animals and humans. As an added bonus, ground pumpkin seeds are also a good source of protein, calcium, zinc, potassium, folic acid, fiber, and niacin, all nutrients that are important for your dog's health.

Other Home Remedies

- **Wheat germ oil.** Some veterinarians suggest you can combine wheat germ oil with ground pumpkin seeds. If you try this remedy, use ¼ teaspoon wheat germ oil plus ¼ teaspoon ground pumpkin seeds for every 10 to 20 pounds of your dog's weight and continue for several weeks.
- **Wormwood.** The herb wormwood (*Artemisia absinthium*) has a long folk history as an herbal fix for intestinal worms and as a digestive tonic. Wormwood contains substances called sesquiterpene lactones, which are believed to weaken the membranes of worms. Herbal worm medications usually con-

tain wormwood. Advocates of wormwood for deworming dogs suggest you give your dog small doses once a week. However, too much wormwood can cause problems with your dog's liver and kidneys.

Suggested Reading/Sources

Alinovi, Cathy, CVM, and Susan Thixton. *Dinner PAWsible: A Cookbook of Healthy Dog & Cat Meals*. CreateSpace Independent Publishing Platform, 2011.

Anne, Jonna, et al. *The Healthy Dog Cookbook: 50 Nutritious & Delicious Recipes Your Dog Will Love*. Neptune City, NJ: TFH Publications, 2008.

Arrowsmith, Claire. *Brain Games for Dogs: Fun Ways to Build a Strong Bond with Your Dog and Provide It with Vital Mental Stimulation*. Surrey, England: Interpet Publishing, 2010.

Brevitz, Betsy, DVM. *The Complete Healthy Dog Handbook: The Definitive Guide to Keeping Your Pet Happy, Healthy & Active*. New York, NY: Workman Publishing Company, 2009.

Eldredge, Debra M., DVM, et al. *Dog Owner's Home Veterinary Handbook*. Hoboken, NJ: Wiley Publishing, 2007.

Fortunato, Lisa. *Everything Cooking for Dogs Book: 150 Quick and Easy Healthy Recipes Your Dog Will Love*. Avon, MA: Adams Media, 2009.

Manteca, X. "Nutrition and Behavior in Senior Dogs." *Topics in Companion Animal Medicine* 26 (1) (February 2011): 33–36.

Martin, Ann N. *Food Pets Die For: Shocking Facts about Pet Food,* 3rd ed. Troutdale, OR: New Sage Press, 2008.

Merck/Merial. *The Merck/Merial Manual for Pet Health: The Complete Pet Health Resource for Your Dog, Cat,*

Horse, or Other Pets—in Everyday Language. Merck, 2007

Messonnier, Shawn, DVM. *The Natural Vet's Guide to Preventing and Treating Arthritis in Dogs and Cats*. Novato, CA: New World Library, 2011.

Messonnier, Shawn, DVM. *Natural Health Bible for Dogs & Cats: Your A–Z Guide to Over 200 Conditions, Herbs, Vitamins, and Supplements*. New York, NY: Three Rivers Press, 2001

Nestle, Marion. *Pet Food Politics: The Chihuahua in the Coal Mine*. Berkeley, CA: University of California Press, 2010.

Nestle, Marion, and Malden Nesheim. *Feed Your Pet Right: The Authoritative Guide to Feeding Your Dog and Cat*. New York, NY: Free Press, 2010.

O'Bryan, Melissa. *Healthy Homemade Dog Food Recipes: The Definitive Guide to All-Natural Meals and Homemade Dog Treats Your Dog Will Love*. CreateSpace Independent Publishing Platform, 2011.

Pitcairn, Richard H., DVM, and Susan H. Pitcairn. *Dr. Pitcairn's New Complete Guide to Natural Health for Dogs and Cats*. Emmaus, PA: Rodale, 2005.

ReBow, Verona, and Jonathan Dune. *Vegetarian Dogs*. http://www.vegetariandogs.com/.

Rivera, Michelle. *Simple Little Vegan Dog Book*. Summertown, TN: Book Publishing Company, 2009.

Tedaldi, Jake, DVM. *What's Wrong with My Dog: A Pet Owner's Guide to 150 Symptoms and What to Do About Them*. Crestline, 2011.

End Notes

Chapter 1

Food and Drug Administration: http://www.fda.gov/Ani malVeterinary/Products/AnimalFoodFeeds/PetFood /UCM2006475.

Dog Training Central: http://www.dog-obedience-training -review.com/homemade-dog-food-recipes.html.

Merck Veterinary Manual: http://www.merckvetmanual .com/mvm/index.jsp?cfile=htm/bc/182902.htm.

National Academy of Sciences: http://dels-old.nas.edu/dels /rpt_briefs/dog_nutrition_final.pdf.

National Research Council: http://dels old.nas.edu/dels/rpt _briefs/dog_nutrition_final.pdf.

National Animal Supplement Council: http://nasc.cc/index .php?option=com_content&task=view&id=29&Itemid=38.

Natural Dog Health Remedies: http://www.natural-dog-health -remedies.com/vitamins-for-dogs.html.

Organic Pet Digest, supplement information: http://www .organic-pet-digest.com/dog-dietary-supplements.html.

Vetinfo.com, vitamin information: http://www.vetinfo.com /dog-multivitamin-guidelines.html.

WebMD dog supplement information: http://pets.webmd .com/dogs/guide/dog-vitamins-and-supplements.

Chapter 2

Association of American Feed Control Officials (AAFCO)

Best Dog Food Guide: http://www.best-dog-food-guide.com /dog-food-manufacturers.html.

Dog Food Project: http://www.dogfoodproject.com/index .php?page=badingredients.

Food and Drug Administration: http://www.fda.gov/Animal Veterinary/Products/AnimalFoodFeeds/PetFood/default .htm.

Whole Dog Journal: http://www.whole-dog-journal.com/is sues/15_6/features/Measuring-Nutritional-Value-in-Dog -Food_20542-1.html.

Chapter 3

Alinovi, Cathy, DVM. Personal communications, May–July 2012.

Dog Channel.com: http://www.dogchannel.com/holistic-dog -care/should-i-feed-my-dog-raw-food.aspx.

Freeman, LM, et al. "Disease Prevalence Among Dogs and Cats in the United States and Australia and Proportions of Dogs and Cats That Receive Therapeutic Diets or Dietary Supplements. *Journal of the American Veterinary Medicine Association* 229 (4) (August 2006): 531–34.

Harbingers of a New Age, information on vegetarian dog food: http://www.vegepet.com/faq_files/Have_any_vet erinarians_recommen.html (accessed July 12, 2012).

Organic Pet Digest: http://www.organic-pet-digest.com/vari able-basic-food.html.

Schlesinger, DP, and DJ Joffe. "Raw Food Diets in Companion Animals: A Critical Review." *Canadian Veterinary Journal* 52 (1) (January 2011): 50–54.

The Whole Dog Journal. "Home-Prepared Dog Food: How

to Make a Balanced Diet." http://www.whole-dog-journal.com/.

Chapter 4

Bierer, TL and LM Bui. "Improvement of Arthritis Signs in Dogs Fed Green-Lipped Mussel (*Perna canaliculus*)." *Journal of Nutrition* 132 (2002): 634S–36S.

Fritsch, DA, et al. "A Multicenter Study of the Effect of Dietary Supplementation with Fish Oil Omega-3 Fatty Acids on Carprofen Dosage in Dogs with Osteoarthritis." *Journal of the American Veterinary Medical Association* 236 (5) (March 2010): 535–39.

Gupta, RC, et al. "Comparative Therapeutic Efficacy and Safety of Type-II Collagen (uc-II), Glucosamine and Chondroitin in Arthritic Dogs: Pain Evaluation by Ground Force Plate." *Journal of Animal Physiology and Animal Nutrition (Berlin)* (May 2011).

Lawson, BR, et al. "Immunomodulation of Murine Collage-Induced Arthritis by N, N-Dimethylglycine and a Preparation of *Perna canaliculus*." *BMC Complementary Alternative Medicine* 7 (June 2007): 20.

McCarthy, G, et al. "Randomised Double-Blind, Positive-Controlled Trial to Assess the Efficacy of Glucosamine Chondroitin Sulfate for the Treatment of Dogs with Osteoarthritis." *Veterinary Journal* (2007).

Messonnier, Shawn, DVM, *The Natural Vet's Guide to Preventing and Treating Arthritis in Dogs and Cats.* 2nd ed. New World Library, 2011.

Pollard, B, et al. "Clinical Efficacy and Tolerance of an Extract of Green-Lipped Mussel (*Perna canaliculus*) in Dogs Presumptively Diagnosed with Degenerative Joint Disease." *New Zealand Veterinary Journal* 54 (3) (June 2006): 114–18.

Roush, JK, et al. "Multicenter Veterinary Practice Assessment of the Effects of Omega-3 Fatty Acids on Osteoarthritis in Dogs." *Journal of the American Veterinary Medical Association* 236 (1) (January 2010): 59–66.

Roush, JK, et al. "Evaluation of the Effects of Dietary Supplementation with Fish Oil Omega-3 Fatty Acids on Weight Bearing in Dogs with Osteoarthritis." *Journal of the American Veterinary Medical Association* 236 (1) (January 2010): 67–73.

Chapter 5

Food allergies: Petmedicine.com. http://www.peteducation.com/article.cfm?c=2+2082&aid=143.

Mueller, RS, et al. "Effect of Omega-3 Fatty Acids on Canine Atopic Dermatitis." *Journal of Small Animal Practice* 45 (6) (June 2004): 293–97.

Chapter 6

Arauio, JA, et al. "Improvement of Short-Term Memory Performance in Aged Beagles by a Nutraceutical Supplement Containing Phosphatidylserine, *Ginkgo biloba*, Vitamin E, and Pyridoxine." *Canadian Veterinary Journal* 49 (4) (April 2008): 379–85.

Cotman, CW, et al. "Brain Aging in the Canine: A Diet Enriched in Antioxidants Reduces Cognitive Dysfunction." *Neurobiology of Aging* 23 (5) (September–October 2002): 809–18.

Dowling, AL, and E Head. "Antioxidants in the Canine Model of Human Aging." *Biochimica et Biophysica Acta* 1822 (5) (May 2002): 685–89.

Pan, Y, et al. "Dietary Supplementation with Medium-Chain TAG Has Long-Lasting Cognition-Enhancing Effects in Aged Dogs." *British Journal of Nutrition* 103 (12) (June 2010): 1746–54.

Reichling, J, et al. "Reduction of Behavioural Disturbances in Elderly Dogs Supplemented with a Standardised Ginkgo

Leaf Extract." *Schweizer Archiv fur Tierheilkunde* 148 (5) (May 2006): 257–63.

Rosado, B, et al. "Effect of Age and Severity of Cognitive Dysfunction on Spontaneous Activity in Pet Dogs." Part 1. Locomotor and Exploratory Behaviour. *Veterinary Journal* (May 2012).

Rosado, B, et al. "Effect of Age and Severity of Cognitive Dysfunction on Spontaneous Activity in Pet Dogs." Part 2. Social Responsiveness. *Veterinary Journal* (May 2012).

Studzinski, CM, et al. "Induction of Ketosis May Improve Mitochondrial Function and Decrease Steady-State Amyloid-Beta Precursor Protein (APP) Levels in the Aged Dog." *Brain Research* 1226 (August 2008): 209–17.

Taha, AY, et al. "Dietary Enrichment with Medium Chain Triglycerides (AC-1203) Elevates Polyunsaturated Fatty Acids in the Parietal Cortex of Aged Dogs: Implications for Treating Age-Related Cognitive Decline." *Neurochemical Research* 34 (9) (September 2009): 1619–25.

Chapter 7

Dental disease: State of Pet Health 2011 Report: http://news.discovery.com/animals/pets-health-cats-dogs-110519.html.

Hudson, JB. "Applications of the Phytomedicine Echinacea Purpurea (Purple Coneflower) in Infectious Diseases." *Journal of Biomedicine & Biotechnology* (2012): 769896.

Prakash, S, et al. "Role of Coenzyme Q10 as an Antioxidant and Bioenergizer in Periodontal Disease." *Indian Journal of Pharmacology* 42 (6) (December 2010): 334–37.

Chapter 8

Hua, Y, et al. "Molecular Mechanisms of Chromium in Alleviating Insulin Resistance." *Journal of Nutritional Biochemistry* 23 (4) (April 2012): 313–19.

Madar, Z, and AH Stark. "New Legume Sources as Therapeutic Agents." *British Journal of Nutrition* 88 Suppl 3 (December 2002): S387–92.

Pitcairn, Richard H., and Susan H. Pitcairn. *Dr. Pitcairn's New Complete Guide to Natural Health for Dogs & Cats.* 3rd ed. Rodale, 2005.

Ribes, G, et al. "Antidiabetic Effects of Subfractions from Fenugreek Seeds in Diabetic Dogs." *Proceedings of the Society for Experimental Biology and Medicine* 182 (2) (June 1986): 159–66.

University of Maryland Medical Center: http://www.umm.edu/altmed/articles/brewers-yeast-000288.htm.

Valette, G, et al. "Hypocholesterolaemic Effect of Fenugreek Seeds in Dogs." *Atherosclerosis* 50 (1) (January 1984): 105–11.

Chapter 9

Herstad, HK, et al. "Effects of a Probiotic Intervention in Acute Canine Gastroenteritis: A Controlled Clinical Trial." *Journal of Small Animal Practice* 51 (1) (January 2010): 34–38.

Kelley, RL, et al. "Clinical Benefits of Probiotic Canine-Derived *Bifidobacterium animalis* Strain AHC7 in Dogs with Acute Idiopathic Diarrhea." *Veterinary Therapy* 10 (3) (Fall 2009): 121–30.

Chapter 10

Natural Dog Health Remedies: http://www.natural-dog-health-remedies.com/dog-ear-infections.html.

Whole Dog Journal: http://www.whole-dog-journal.com/issues/7_10/features/Canine-Ear_15661-1.html.

Chapter 11

Hink, WF, and BJ Fee. "Toxicity of D-Limonene, the Major Component of Citrus Peel Oil, to All Life Stages of the Cat Flea, *Ctenocephalides felis* (Siphonaptera: Pulicidae)." *Journal of Medical Entomology* 23 (4) (July 1986): 400–404.

Schmahl, G, et al. "The Efficacy of Neem Seed Extracts (Tresan, MiteStop) on a Broad Spectrum of Pests and Parasites." *Parasitology Research* 107 (2) (July 2010): 261–69.

Smith, CA. "Searching for Safe Methods of Flea Control." *Journal of the American Veterinary Medical Association* 206 (8) (April 1995): 1137–43.

Chapter 12

Brown, SA, et al. "Effects of Dietary Polyunsaturated Fatty Acid Supplementation in Early Renal Insufficiency in Dogs." *Journal of Laboratory Clinical Medicine* 135 (3) (March 2000): 275–86.

Brown, SA, et al. "Beneficial Effects of Chronic Administration of Dietary Omega-3 Polyunsaturated Fatty Acids in Dogs with Renal Insufficiency." *Journal of Laboratory and Clinical Medicine* 131 (5) (May 1998): 447–55.

Fassett, RG, et al. "Omega-3 Polyunsaturated Fatty Acids in the Treatment of Kidney Disease." *American Journal of Kidney Diseases* 56 (4) (October 2010): 728–42.

Mori, TA, et al. "The Effects of [Omega]3 Fatty Acids and Coenzyme Q10 on Blood Pressure and Heart Rate in Chronic Kidney Disease: A Randomized Controlled Trial." *Journal of Hypertension* 27 (9) (September 2009): 1863–72.

Pitcairn, Richard H., and Susan H. Pitcairn. *Dr. Pitcairn's New Complete Guide to Natural Health for Dogs and Cats.* 3rd ed. Rodale, 2005.

Song, H, et al. "Investigation of Urinary Interleukin-6 Level in Chronic Renal Failure Patients and the Influence of *Rheum palmatum* in Treating It." *Zhongguo Zhong Xi Yi Jie H Z Zhi* 20 (2) (February 2000): 107–9.

Xiao, W, et al. "Summarization of the Clinical and Laboratory Study on the Rhubarb in Treating Chronic Renal Failure." *Zhongguo Zhong Yao Za Zhi* 27 (4) (April 2002): 241–44.

Chapter 13

American Pet Products Manufacturers Association: 2010 US Pet Population.

Armstrong, PJ. "Managing Weight Loss in Dogs and Cats (Proceedings)." CVC in Kansas City Proceedings, Aug 1, 2010. http://veterinarycalendar.dvm360.com/avhc/article/articleDetail.jsp?id=746671&pageID=1&sk=&date= (accessed July 2, 2012).

Chen, SC, et al. "Effect of Conjugated Linoleic Acid Supplementation on Weight Loss and Body Fat Composition in a Chinese Population." *Nutrition* 28 (5) (May 2012): 559–65.

DeLany, JP, and DB West. "Changes in Body Composition with Conjugated Linoleic Acid." *Journal of the American College of Nutrition* 19 (2000): 487S–493S.

DogAware.com. http://www.dogaware.com/articles/wdjlowfatdietsamples.html.

Kurzman, ID, et al. "The Effect of Dehydroepiandrosterone Combined with a Low-Fat Diet in Spontaneously Obese Dogs: A Clinical Trial." *Obesity Research* 6 (1) (January 1998): 20–28.

Kurzman, ID, et al. "Reduction in Body Weight and Cholesterol in Spontaneously Obese Dogs by Dehydroepiandrosterone." *International Journal of Obesity* 14 (2) (February 1990): 95–104.

MacEwen, EG, and ID Kurzman. "Obesity in the Dog: Role

of the Adrenal Steroid Dehydroepiandrosterone (DHEA)." *Journal of Nutrition* 121 (11 Suppl) (November 1991): S51–55.

Rand, JS, et al. "Diet in the Prevention of Diabetes and Obesity in Companion Animals." *Asia Pacific Journal of Clinical Nutrition* 12 Suppl (2003): S6.

Whole Dog Journal Low fat diet: http://www.whole-dog -journal.com/issues/11_12/features/Healthy-Low-Fat -Dog-Foods_16088-1.html.

Chapter 14

Axelsson, I. "Honey, Not Dextromethorphan, Was Better Than No Treatment for Nocturnal Cough in Children with Upper Respiratory Infections." *Evidence Based Medicine* 13 (4) (August 2008): 106.

Schwartz, Cheryl, DVM. *Four Paws, Five Directions: A Guide to Chinese Medicine for Cats and Dogs.* Celestial Arts, 1996.

Warren, MD, and WO Cooper. "Honey Improves Cough in Children Compared to No Treatment." *Journal of Pediatrics* 152 (5) (May 2008): 739–40.

Chapter 15

Schwartz, Cheryl, DVM. *Four Paws, Five Directions: A Guide to Chinese Medicine for Cats and Dogs.* Celestial Arts, 1996.

Pet Wave. Urinary tract infections: http://www.petwave.com /Dogs/Dog-Health-Center/Kidney-and-Urinary-Tract -Disorders/Urinary-Tract-Infections/Causes.aspx.

Chapter 16

Haniadka, R, et al. "*Zingiber officinale* (ginger) as an Anti-Emetic in Cancer Chemotherapy: A Review." *Journal of*

Alternative & Complementary Medicine 18 (5) (May 2012): 440–44.

Herstad, HK, et al. "Effects of a Probiotic Intervention in Acute Canine Gastroenteritis: A Controlled Clinical Trial." *Journal of Small Animal Practice* 51 (1) (January 2010): 34–38.

Williamson, KK, et al. "Efficacy of Famotidine for the Prevention of Exercise-Induced Gastritis in Racing Alaskan Sled Dogs." *Journal of Veterinary Internal Medicine* 21 (5) (September–October 2007): 924–27.

Williamson, KK, et al. "Efficacy of Omeprazole Versus High-Dose Famotidine for Prevention of Exercise-Induced Gastritis in Racing Alaskan Sled Dogs." *Journal of Veterinary Internal Medicine* 24 (2) (April–May 2010): 285–88.

Chapter 17

Ayaz, E, et al. "Evaluation of the Anthelmentic Activity of Garlic (*Allium sativum*) in Mice Naturally Infected with *Aspiculuris tetraptera*." *Recent Patents on Anti-infective Drug Discovery* 3 (2) (June 2008): 149–52.

Appendix

20+ Foods and Beverages Dogs Should Not Consume

Alcohol: You may have seen people give their dogs a beer, but alcohol in any form—beer, wine, spirits, and foods that contain alcohol—may harm your dog. Even small amounts can cause diarrhea, vomiting, breathing difficulties, central nervous system depression, coordination problems, and even death.

Avocados: Resist the temptation to share guacamole dip with your pooch. Although a tiny amount of avocado fruit may not be harmful to your dog, large amounts may be toxic. That's because avocados contain a substance called persin. If you have any avocado plants growing in areas where your dog has access, make sure he stays away from them, because the seeds, leaves, and bark are also toxic.

Bones and Fat: Do not give your dog cooked bones of any type, because they can easily splinter and cause lots of problems, ranging from broken teeth to punctured digestive tract. Raw bones are spongy, but accidents can still occur. When you trim the fat from your steak, don't toss it to your dog. Both cooked and uncooked fat can cause pancreatitis in dogs.

Caffeine: Small amounts of caffeine from coffee, tea, cocoa, colas, stimulant drinks (e.g., Red Bull), and medications that contain caffeine can cause caffeine poisoning, which is characterized by bleeding, fits, muscle tremors, heart palpitations, rapid breathing and restlessness. In large quantities, caffeine can be fatal.

Cat food: If you have cats and your dog occasionally feasts on the cat food, don't panic. However, cat food contains very high protein and fats that are not recommended for dogs.

Chocolate: You may know of a dog who ate chocolate and nothing happened, but don't take that chance. Chocolate contains theobromine, theophylline, sugar, and caffeine, and it can cause vomiting, diarrhea, excessive thirst, abnormal heart rhythms, tremors, seizures, and even death. The most dangerous chocolates are dark chocolate and unsweetened baking chocolate, but others, including white chocolate, are also dangerous.

Garlic and onions: There is confusion and some disagreement about the safety of garlic for dogs. Garlic is recommended in small amounts to treat a variety of health problems, and when used as directed it can be beneficial. However, large amounts of garlic or onions or eating small amounts of either one over a long period of time may cause symptoms, such as anemia, vomiting, breathlessness, and loss of appetite.

Grapes, raisins, and currants: These seemingly tasty treats for dogs can cause kidney failure, and experts are not certain why. However, even a small amount of either food can cause repeated vomiting (an early sign) followed by lethargy and depression.

Iron supplements: Supplements for people that contain iron can damage the lining of the digestive system and may also have a negative impact on the liver and kidneys.

Macadamia nuts: Keep your dog away from your nuts and macadamia cookies. Just a few raw or roasted macadamia nuts can make your dog ill and experience muscle tremors, weakness or paralysis of the hind legs, vomiting, and rapid heart rate.

Milk and milk products: Both milk and milk-based foods such as ice cream may cause diarrhea and are also associated with food allergies, which can show up as itching and scratching. However, small amounts of yogurt (which contains healthful probiotics) and some cheeses such as farmer cheese are accepted by many dogs.

Peaches, persimmons, and plums: You can give your dog the flesh of these fruits, but not the seeds or pits. Persimmon seeds can cause inflammation of the small intestine or intestinal obstruction in dogs, while peach and plum pits also can cause obstruction. In addition, plum and peach pits contain cyanide.

Raw eggs: Giving your dog raw eggs presents two possible problems. One is that raw egg whites contain an enzyme that disrupts the absorption of the B vitamin biotin. The second problem is the possibility of food poisoning from salmonella or E. coli, both of which are frequently found in eggs.

Raw fish and meat: Although some people advocate a raw food diet for dogs, raw fish and meat can contain harmful bacteria that can even prove to be deadly for your dog.

Raw potatoes: Cooked potatoes are fine, but don't give raw potatoes or any potato plants to your dog, including access to potatoes in a garden.

Salt: Excessive salt in the form of salty foods (e.g., chips, pretzels) can result in abnormal thirst and urination, vomiting, diarrhea, elevated body temperature, tremors, and seizures.

Sugar: Too much sugar can lead to obesity, diabetes, and dental problems.

Xylitol: This artificial sweetener is found in candies, gum, baked goods, and some diet foods, and it is not recommended for dogs. That's because it can trigger an increase in insulin levels and cause your dog's blood glucose levels to drop. It also may contribute to liver failure. Symptoms associated with ingesting xylitol include vomiting, loss of coordination, and lethargy.

Sources of Information on Dog Food, Dog Treats, and Supplements

The following is a representative list only and is no way an endorsement of any company or organization.

Association for Pet Obesity Prevention (APOP)
This association has developed an online pet weight translator that helps pet parents determine if their dog is overweight.
http://www.petobesityprevention.com/pet-weight-translator/

ConsumerLab.com
Provides reviews of a wide range of supplements. Primarily a site for human supplements, but it does have some pet products. Only some information is free; there is a subscription price as well.
http://www.consumerlab.com/

Dog Vitamin Reviews
Reviews of a wide range of dog vitamins and supplements.
http://www.dogvitaminreviews.com/

Dog Food Advisor
Provides several different lists of dog foods for you to compare, including grain free, low-fat, and an overall list.
http://www.dogfoodadvisor.com/

The Dog Food Project
Comprehensive information on dog food labeling and the dog food industry, including dog food ingredients to avoid.

http://www.dogfoodproject.com/index.php?page=label
info101

Dog Food Scoop
A dog food comparison chart listing approximately one hundred dog food brands, most of which are from small companies.
http://www.dogfoodscoop.com/dog-food-comparison.html

National Academy of Sciences
Nutritional information on dog food.
http://dels-old.nas.edu/dels/rpt_briefs/dog_nutrition_final.pdf

National Research Council
Nutritional information on dog food.
http://dels-old.nas.edu/dels/rpt_briefs/dog_nutrition_final.pdf

National Animal Supplement Council
An organization whose members are manufacturers of animal health supplements and who strive to improve the quality of these products sold for cats, dogs, and other companion animals.
http://nasc.cc/

Truth about Pet Food
Comprehensive (and disturbing) information about the pet food industry.
http://www.truthaboutpetfood.com/articles/disturbing-%28and-illegal%29-fda-compliance-policies.html

Vegetarian Dogs.com
Provides information on dog food, nutrition, supplements, exercise, and care of vegetarian and vegan dogs.
http://www.vegetarianDogs.com/